Prescription For Life

by

Edward A. Taub, M.D.

Commendations by
Norman Cousins
Author of *Anatomy of an Illness*

Ron Pion, M.D.
Founder of Hospital Satellite Network
Originator of Group I Medical

Revised 2nd edition

You will hardly know
Who I am or what I mean,
But I shall be good health
to you nevertheless,
And filter and fiber your blood.

Failing to find me at first
keep encouraged.
Missing me one place search another.
I stop somewhere waiting for you.

–LEAVES OF GRASS
Walt Whitman

Commendation

...A work of extraordinary merit...
The wise physician today recognizes that the physiological and psychological resources of the patient are an important part of a total strategy of treatment along with the best that modern medical science has to offer. Edward Taub's book is an up-to-date guide on putting the patient's own resources to work. In so doing, he makes full use of the latest research in the concept of the patient-physician partnership.

Norman Cousins
Author: Anatomy of an Illness

Commendation

I first encountered Dr. Ed Taub when I returned to Southern California some nine years ago. He was engaged then, as he is now, in his quest to find suitable environments in which he might more efficiently guide others in their promotion of health and prevention of disease.

Like all good teachers, Ed continues to grow as a consequence of the students and patients with whom he interacts. His teaching skills improve; his curriculum remains challenging and varied; and he demonstrates a remarkable ability to imbue others with the adventure of search and discovery.

There are those champions of traditional Western medical philosophy that hold tenaciously to the belief that the mind has no influence over physical illness. Dr. Taub on the other hand, schooled in this same philosophy, has observed too many instances of scientifically 'unexplained' healing. Like other good medical historians, he chronicles these instances, and seeks to understand them by opening his mind to the possibility of the potential for spiritual cure.

The recent emergence of research in the field of neuropeptides may soon shed light on the mechanisms that "link" mind and body. Newer studies of this class of chemicals have provided interesting data suggesting the role they play in connecting the brain with the immune system, and other body systems. For example, the group of opioid peptides, endorphins among them, are responsible for that wonderful feeling of accomplishment after hard work, and the joy experienced after eating, or during and after participation in sex.

Further investigation of the relationship between the body's hormonal systems, the neuropeptides, and our emotions, may shed new light on the powerful ways meditation and visualization can augment current medical practice. It would seem foolish to offer these powerful alternatives to but a small select group of patients 'failed' by modern Western medicine, i.e. those with end stage cancer, or other 'terminal' disease. I would prefer that physicians consider offering these and other practices to their pediatric and young adult patients before they were to become ill. Certainly, a 'scientific' approach can be included so that, that which works is distinguishable from that which doesn't, and the physician can support the credo of 'primum non nocere', - physician do no harm.

Integrative Medicine is an emerging discipline that can be utilized by health care professionals and the patients they are called upon to serve.

Ron Pion M.D.
Clinical Professor of Obstetrics
and Gynecology, U.C.L.A.

Dedication

Lovingly for Sathya Sai Baba

Integrative Medicine is an adjunct to the traditional disease-repair system. It is not the intent of the author to diagnose and prescribe and he therefore does not assume any responsibility for your health care. The author's intent is only to offer health information to help you cooperate with your doctor in your mutual quest for health.

Important Note to the Reader

The meditation therapy tape accompanying this book is an integral part of **Prescription For Life.** It is extremely important for you to use the tape to quiet your thoughts for a successful journey.

The tape features a new scientific technology called brain synchronization. The special combination of subtle tones and frequencies balance both the right and left hemispheres of your brain and induce deep relaxation. For that reason do not listen while driving or operating a machine. For best results be sure to use headphones. All the messages and information that you hear will be absorbed on deep inner levels.

Table of Contents

COMMENDATIONS iii, v
ACKNOWLEDGEMENTS xv
FOREWORD xix
INFORMATION FOR PHYSICIANS xxv

I   THE DILEMMA OF THE SICK
    AND TIRED 1
    Tender Loving Care 1
    Psychoneuroimmunology and
    Integrative Medicine 8
    Diagnostic Entrapment 12

II THE WORRIED WELL AND THE
    WALKING WOUNDED 19
    Invitation to Wellness 19
    What Wellness Is 29
    Illness Inducing Thoughts 30
    Sick Business 42
    Miracle Healings 44
    Thought Energy 47

III THE ENDANGERED MIND 53
    Reverence For Life 53
    A Little History and a Lot
    of Technology 57
    Beginnings of Integrative Medicine ... 60
    A New Kind of Practice 63
    Wellness Measurements 71
    The Taub Response-Ability Scale 76

Your Response-Ability Quotient.... 78
What It Means................... 78

IV THE "S FACTOR"................ 85
   Smouldering Slow Stress Syndrome... 85
   Mind Cancer 90
   Templates of Disease 91
   Cancer is a Genetic Disease 98
   Life Promoters.................. 99

V UNDERSTANDING ENERGY..... 109
   Foreign Energy 114

VI I LACK LOVE (I-L-L) 129

VII "THE THINKER"................ 145
   Be Happy Not Right............. 145
   Caution: Ego at Work 152
   Media and World View 155
   Stress and Disease 157

VIII VOYAGE TO WELLNESS........ 165
   Ingredient One: Quieting the Mind ... 170
   Ingredient Two: Exercise.......... 187
   Ingredient Three: Energy Nutrition ... 194
   Ingredient Four: Addiction 203
   Ingredient Five: Self-Safety........ 207
   Ingredient Six: Lovingness......... 209
   Ingredient Seven: Ethical Living.... 213

IX YOUR WELLNESS CONTRACT... 217

X   THE LAST HURDLE.............. 231

XI WEEK BY WEEK OVERVIEW 237

    CONCLUSION 251
    EPILOGUE 255
    BIBLIOGRAPHY-GENERAL 261
    BIBLIOGRAPHY-
    PSYCHONEUROIMMUNOLOGY...... 267
    ABOUT THE AUTHOR.............. 273

Acknowledgements

The ideas that gave birth to Integrative Medicine were synthesized from the work and teachings of the initial Advisory Board of the Foundation for Health Awareness.

Sidney Adler, M.D.
Robert Aldrich, M.D.
Harold Bloomfield, M.D.
Paul Brenner, M.D.
Barbara Brown, Ph.D.
Richard Byrne, Ph.D.
Norman Cousins
Merlin DuVal, M.D.
Joel Elkes, M.D.
Marilyn Ferguson
Phyllis Gallagher, R.N.,J.D.
Cal Hetrick
Barbara Marx Hubbard
Max Kamen, D.O.

David Law, M.D.
Lee Kearney
Eugene Levin, M.D.
Stanley Matek
Douglas Mayer
Ashley Montague, Ph.D.
Ron Pion, M.D.
Grayce Roessler, R.N.,Ph.D.
Albert Rosenfeld
Serina Taub, R.N., Ph.D.
Lanny Taub, M.D.
Jon Thie, D.C.
Tim Twombly, D.C.
Olga Worrall

Other individuals have devoted their lives to scientific excellence and spiritual and moral balance; they have contributed to the birth of Integrative Medicine.

Randolph Ballantine, M.D.
Martin Baren, M.D.
Herbert Benson, M.D.
Joan Borysenko, Ph.D.
Warren Brandli, D.D.S.
David Bressler, Ph.D.
Rick Carlson
Ram Dass
Harvey Diamond
Marilyn Diamond
Larry Dossey, M.D.
Tom Ferguson, M.D.
Stanley Greben, M.D.
Vic Greco, M.D.
David Harris
John Hislop, Ph.D.
Jean Houston, Ph.D.
Rick Ingrasci, M.D.
Daniel Ivler, Ph.D.
Dennis Jaffe, Ph.D.
John James, M.D.
Gerald Jampolsky, M.D.
Brugh Joy, M.D.
Charles Kleeman, M.D.
Elizabeth Kubler-Ross, M.D.
Steven Locke, M.D.

Robert Mendelsohn, M.D.
Emmett Miller, M.D.
Frederick O'Connell, M.D.
Dean Ornish, M.D.
Irving Oyle, M.D.
William Parker, Ph.D.
Scott Peck, M.D.
Kenneth Pellitier, Ph.D.
Karl Pribram, M.D.
Julius Richmond, M.D.
Clara Riley, Ph.D.
Jonas Salk, M.D.
Samuel Sandweiss, M.D.
Hans Selye, M.D.
Ken Sereno, Ph.D.
Norman Shealy, M.D.
Bernie Siegel, M.D.
O. Carl Simonton, M.D.
Tom Sinclair, M.D.
John Smith, M.D.
Lendon Smith, M.D.
George Solomon, M.D.
Jacques Souadjian, M.D.
John Travis, M.D.
Lawrence Weed, M.D.
Paul Wehrle, M.D.
Andrew Weil, M.D.

Many individuals supported my work during it's birthing pains: Anneli Taub, Judy Hill, Marc Taub, Valerie Creekmore, Joe Garma, Karen Maroney, Rae Lynn Price, Fred Adickes, Ed Doyle, Mike Mesenbrink, Jim Crooks, Woody Anderson, Thomas Standish Ph.D., Walter Jayasinghe, M.D., Eileen Lewis, Henry and Eve Rose, and Homer and Wilmaglen Bergren: there was Serina Taub's major influence, a season of Lisa Tracy's work, the communications skills that Lora Taub lovingly shared with me, and the outstanding editing of Patti Breitman. Always, in all ways, there was my brother Lanny, my parents, my friends, Ron and Sue Myers, and my mentor Cready Irwin.

I was especially inspired by Julius Richmond, M.D., Paul Wehrle, M.D., Charles Kleeman, M.D., Merlin DuVal, M.D., Hans Selye, M.D., Jonas Salk, M.D., and Albert Schweitzer.

I owe special thanks to John F. Holman, the President of the American Wellness Association, for his courage, direction and concept of the "S Factor".

Foreword
by
Harvey and Marilyn Diamond
Authors: *Fit For Life*

During the last decades of the Twentieth Century, we as a people began coming to a new awareness about our bodies. It is a simple and obvious awareness and it is mind boggling that we lived without it for so long.

What is this new consciousness? It is that our bodies belong to us and that our health is our responsibility. Having relinquished that precious control over our bodies to a health care system accustomed to dictating to us, we now seek to reclaim our autonomy. We have learned what the consequences can be having lived without it.

For centuries we have endured the pervasive philosophy that our health was out of our control. Children of a species that survived and flourished for hundreds of thousands of years in harmony with itelf and its environment, we were taught to turn our backs on our instinctive ability to survive and be well as we had done for the eons of pre-history. We were persuaded to rely totally on outside forces and agents of healing to maintain our health.

From an intuitive awareness that our bodies were capable of healing themselves, we were led further and further down the path of dependence and non-responsibility to a place where, until recently, we no longer participated even minimally in decisions about how to care for our bodies. But the winds of change bring us enlightenment we so desperately seek in the form of books and works such as the one you, dear reader, now hold in your hand. Hold it lovingly, cherish it, and take it seriously, for Edward A. Taub has written here for you a *prescription*, a strategy that you can embrace to participate fully and, if you wish, independently, in the care of your body and the restoration of your health. In so doing, Dr. Taub joins a new breed of health care advocates, guides, and specialists, openly speaking to you for the first time in over a century, bringing to you a free flow of ideas and philosophies about what *you* can do to be in full control of your health, working *with* rather than against the *innate healing ability of your own body*.

Dr. Taub is opening new doors. As a licensed physician, for twenty-five years in general practice, he has taken the time to investigate the major philosophies of health care inside as well as *outside* the medical model. He has embraced and acknowledged the unbroken thread of philosophy that runs through all natural approaches to health care, that *healing is done by the body as a conscious living system* and that the responsibility of the practitioner is to "first, do no harm" and second, work with the body's resources to heal itself.

Dr. Taub bridges a gap and opens a new frontier for all health practitioners and health seekers. In uncomplicated, lay terms, with an eloquence, clarity and compassion seldom found in medical texts he brings to the public a loving way to bridge the gap to the future.

We have known Doctor Taub intimately as a friend, supporter, and advisor since the early part of this decade. His dedication to your health has since that time driven him to hold fast to his ideals. His living vision has been that there is a new and better direction in which medical practitioners can and must go and that it falls on his shoulders to break new ground and lead in that direction.

This book is a gift of wisdom and practicality to the lay person as well as to the specialist. It reaffirms that which cannot be reaffirmed often enough: that we have *the right* to take care of our bodies, that we *can* take care of our bodies, and that health, vibrant, glorious health, is the birthright of each and every one of us.

Information For Physicians

INFORMATION FOR PHYSICIANS*

Integrative Medicine is a paradigm of self-empowerment for physicians and patients. The practice of Integrative Medicine is a synthesis of western scientific medicine, eastern, oriental, ayurvedic and folkloric medicine, with the addition of a spiritual dimension that we can no longer afford to ignore.

Integrative Medicine is not derivative. Rather, it is representative of a new format of self-health care for patients that is based on the following paradigm: **health is utimately determined by personal responsibility, self value and reverence for life.**

This medical paradigm is integrative in it's *function*. It is based on:

(1) primum non nocere (firstly doing no harm),

(2) supporting remedies that are less invasive,

(3) seeking less costly more natural alternatives to care.

*Although I personally and professionally address my fellow physicians, this information is entirely appropriate for *all* health care professionals.

This medical paradigm is integrative in *intent*. It insists on:

(1) placing patients in the role of having clear responsibility for their own attitudes, lifestyles and habits,

(2) calling for patients to assume full partnership with their physicians for health maintenance and care.

Integrative Medicine offers a complementary diagnostic and treatment program for both the general and specialty physician to upgrade their knowledge and skill and to become more effective in this late twentieth century when stress has become the new national "virus." This new medical paradigm combines high tech with high touch and is easily entered into through the simple acceptance that our patients are a combination of body, mind, and spirit.

Stress, defined as our harmful *response and reaction* to events and circumstances, is so rampant and epidemic that its role in the premature emergence of disease can no longer be ignored or merely paid lip service to. Sir William Osler saw this coming at the beginning of this century when he declared that the cure of tuberculosis depended more on what a patient had in his head than in his chest.

It is no longer tenable for the modern clinician to eliminate the stress factor as a major etiological factor and primary therapeutic consideration in virtually all disease; we would be toying with our patients' futures. All clinical physicians basically know this to be true—yet we have been hampered by the lack of format to proceed with—a therapeutic armentarium for care. Integrative Medicine enables us to proceed.

Integrative Medicine owes itself to the work and the minds of the individuals who made up the advisory board of the Foundation for Health Awareness. All of the Advisors have been listed in the acknowledgements to this book. I am particularly indebted to the following individuals who formed the initial Advisory Council. I have listed their credentials from the early part of this decade when Integrative Medicine began emerging from their ideas.

JOEL ELKES, M.D., Distinguished Service Professor and former Director of the Department of Psychiatry and Behavioral Sciences at Johns-Hopkins University.

MARILYN FERGUSON, Author, *Aquarian Conspiracy.* Editor, *Brain Mind Bulletin.*

STANLEY MATEK, President, American Public Health Association.

ASHLEY MONTAGUE, Ph.D., Chairman of the Department of Medical Anthopology, Princeton University.

RON PION, M.D., Clinical Professor of Obstetrics and Gynecology, U.C.L.A. Founder of Hospital Satellite Network.

GRACE ROESSLER, R.N., Ph.D., Coordinator, Continuing Education, Goldenwest University.

ALBERT ROSENFELD, Consultant, March of Dimes. Former Science Editor, *Saturday Review and Time-Life Inc.*

LANNY TAUB, M.D., Assistant Clinical Professor, University of California at Irvine.

SERINA TAUB R.N., Ph.D., Founder of the Institute for Health Facilitation.

Hundreds of thousands of individuals have been taught the principles of Integrative Medicine and are now aware of their ability to help themselves stay well. They are also aware of their responsibility for helping themselves get well once they have become sick. As a clinician, able to gauge the extent of my patients' well-being, I am quite certain that this awareness creates significant differences in the ways that people think, act and behave.

A well designed retrospective study is of course necessary to demonstrate long-term results. Perhaps the changes and additions that may be needed in the therapeutic armamentarium presented in this book will come from you.

Please feel free to use parts of this book with your patients - i.e., The Wellness Contract, The Responsibility Scale, etc. In return, please consider sending copies of completed contracts and questionaires as well as your clinical impressions of results to: The American Wellness Association, 3030 Bridgeway, Sausalito, California, 94965. Perhaps your observations will help to build the cornerstone for a preventatively designed and wellness-oriented health insurance system.

This book is written in very simple language in order to be easily understood by patients from all walks of life and educational levels. The book has been written to be used along with a meditation therapy audio cassette tape. The purpose of the tape is to help quiet the mind of the reader to reduce the effects of stress, increase retention of knowledge, and allow the body's own disease repair systems to operate more effectively. The tape features a new scientific technology called brain synchronization. The brain synchronization process consists of a special combination of subtle tones and frequencies that balance both the right and left hemispheres of the brain and induce deep relaxation. For best results the tape should be listened to with headphones.

I have found the brain synchronizing sound technology and the guided meditation therapy on the accompanying tape to be extremely effective. It quiets the mind and induces the meditative state—a state that I define quite simply as stillness of thought. Again, valid measuring techniques need to be developed, but the brain synchronizing sound process on the tape literally "meditates" the listener; the thinking, fearing, worrying part of the brain is suppressed and the intuitive, imaginative, creative part is enhanced. Endorphins flow, options are seen more clearly, and *self empowerment* occurs—the ability to move forward or to go forth in a previously hostile or confusing environment.

One of my advisors, a brilliant and accomplished individual, literally has perfect pitch. He is also a completely linear thinker who nevertheless after listening to the brain synchronizing tones and frequencies and meditation, told me, "I hear God."

Plato one of the smartest and most revered mortals of his day, lamented the fact that physicians insisted on treating patients as if their mind, body and soul were separate. The foundation of Integrative Medicine is that we are body, mind and spirit. Just as water is also steam and ice.

Mind is the quality or the entity that regulates the entire organism—the neuro-endocrinological-immunological coordinator present wherever regulated cellular metabolism takes place, which is everywhere.

Spirit is the quality or entity of the human organism that searches for love and for meaning. It is an indefinable essence in the human being that reaches out to encompass goodness and wisdom and a concept of God.

Integrative Medicine recognizes all these as facets of a human being, and the need to treat these aspects to achieve a state of personal wellness.

Socrates was Plato's teacher. Socrates reminded the so-called authorities of how very ignorant they were of their own ignorance. His life was taken for his reminders. We physicians, part of a proud and glorious profession now becoming rather frayed around the edges, must no longer continue to ignore *our* ignorance of what lies beyond our scientifically based, linear thought processes: Man's search for meaning, his unflagging quest for love and his aspirations for integrity. These are not measureable qualities yet they make up the most powerful factor that we as physicians can use to empower our patients to become well and stay well—*because in this day and age our patients' health is generally determined by personal responsibility, self value and reverence for life.* The empowerment of nature's healing force, the stimulation of homeo-stasis, the glorification of what Hippocrates called the vis medicatrix naturae, must be our goal. We were taught to do no less than this in medical school, and that's what Integrative Medicine is about.

HOW DOES A PHYSICIAN PRACTICE INTEGRATIVE MEDICINE?

Simply by working within the following paradigm and belief system:

1. Illnesses begin primarily in our patients' minds.
2. Our highest duty is enhancing, the *vis mediatrix naturae*, the healing ability of our patients.
3. The body and mind have the potential to reverse any disease as long as tissue death has not occurred.
4. Food is either live and full of vitality or dead and embalmed.
5. Regular exercise of some sort is a pre-requisite for good health.
6. Everything in moderation, (including moderation).
7. Never place blame or stimulate guilt in patients no matter what they do or refuse to do.
8. Be tolerant and have a basic awareness of Eastern, Oriental, Aryuvedic, Homeopathic, Chiropractic and Osteopathic Medicine.
9. Remember that approximately 80% of prescribed drugs work as well as a placebo.
10. Remember our medical school teaching to never cease in our efforts to avoid surgery, hospital-

ization and radiation unless clearly and absolutely
necessary.

WHAT DO YOU TELL YOUR PATIENTS?

Tell them you want to be their "Wellness
doctor" as well as their sickness doctor. Then
spend the necessary time to do it well.

PERSONAL WELLNESS SYSTEM

The *Prescription For Life* book and its accompanying audiocassette tape are one part of a complete *Personal Wellness System*. The system had been designed by Dr. Taub and the American Wellness Association (AWA).

The complementary parts of the system are: 1) Disease Specific Audiocassettes; 2) the *7-Day Stress Relief System*; 3) The *Fitness Option* book, audiocassette, and videotape; and 4) Dr. Taub's *Voyage to Wellness* lecture series.

DISEASE SPECIFIC AUDIOCASSETTES

The first step toward curing a disease is understanding the disease itself. Accordingly, working in conjunction with the AWA, Dr. Taub has created a series of disease specific audiocassettes that begin like a visit to your health care practitioner.

On Side A of each 60 minute audiocassette, Dr. Taub discusses your disease from a medical perspective in order to help you understand and visualize your illness. Side B of each audiocassette contains a *Directed Relaxation Therapy* session designed to address each specific disease. Using it, you will experience a deep state of relaxation that will help your body's natural healing forces to work to their fullest capacity.

Both sides of each audiocassette contains the patented *Brain Synchronization* process that is utilized on the *Prescription For Life* audio cassette that accompanies this book. The process combines subtle musical tones and frequencies to bring the right and left hemispheres of the brain into balance.

In 1981, Dr. Roger Sperry received the Nobel prize for demonstrating that the right and left hemispheres of the brain perform very different functions. The right side influences the creative process. When you write a song, read a poem or paint a picture, you are predominately exercising the right hemisphere of the brain. The left side influences the analytical, rational functions. When you are using a computer for analysis, balancing a checkbook, or compiling a shopping list, you are predominately utilizing the left hemisphere of the brain.

By bringing both hemispheres of the brain into focused balance, the *Brain Synchronization* process induces a state of deep relaxation and helps stimulate your body's natural healing forces. The disease specific audiocassettes currently available include: Backache, Weight Loss, Insomnia, Cancer, Alcohol, Smoking, Drug Abuse, Health Rejuvenation, and Childhood Illnesses (for parents and children). The price is $11.95 each.

THE 7-DAY STRESS RELIEF SYSTEM

The **7-Day Stress Relief System** developed by Edward A. Taub, M.D., and the American Wellness Association is an eight-audiocassette library designed to help control stress and worry that results from our current American lifestyle. Each of the audiocassette tapes utilize both the patented *Brain Synchronization* process and the *Directed Relaxation Therapy (DRT)* technique.

The first tape in the audiocassette library discusses stress from a medical perspective and gives you a *Personal Wellness Prescription* that is easy to implement into your life. The remaining seven tapes contain unique *Directed Relaxation Therapy* sessions, each building on the foundation laid by the prior tape, that are to be used over a seven day period. At the end of seven days, the cumulative effects of this system will make a lasting, positive impact on reducing the harmful effects of stress and increasing the ability of your body to generate its own natural healing forces.

The system is designed to be used whenever you need its help in dealing with stress. The system has proven to be effective in reducing stress and relieving dis-ease. The price of the *Stress Relief System* is $99.95.

THE FITNESS OPTION

Today, physical exercise is widely recognized as an excellent method of stress relief. However, it is not widely understood that many types of less strenuous exercise can be done by virtually anyone and produce the same level of stress reduction as running or aerobics.

The Fitness Option book, audiocassette and videotape teach a 5-week exercise curriculum that reduces stress through stretch and flex exercises, breathing techniques and deep relaxation skills. The course incorporates Western and Eastern psychotherapy and relaxation methods.

The book was written by Valerie O'Hara, Ph.D., who has been teaching stress management techniques for the past 18 years. The book is an approved textbook at the University of California and provides numerous graphic examples of each exercise presented.

Each week's instructions provide practical, step by step, guidance on incorporating the skills learned in the program into your lifestyle. The program was created specifically to help you manage stress without it becoming a time consuming endeavor. One day at a time, you can integrate tension-relieving techniques into your daily routine. Soon, you will approach optimal health as you stretch to your fullest potential.

Each week's routine begins with a different breathing exercise that effectively focuses your attention in the moment. The breathing exercises relieve negative, draining emotions such as fear and anxiety, and in their place allow a calm revitalization to occur. After the breathing exercises, each weekly routine features physical exercises to release muscular tension. Thereafter, you are provided with deep relaxation procedures, including the widely heraled *Jacobson Progressive Muscle Relaxation Technique.*

The audiocassette and videotape make it easy for you to follow along with Dr. O'Hara through each of the exercises and techniques. The program is designed for people of all ages, and does not require you to be athletic. All that is required is a desire to reduce the stress level in your life and to get well. The price of the *Fitness Option* book, audiocassette and videotape is $49.95.

VOYAGE TO WELLNESS LECTURE SERIES

Since 1985, Dr. Taub has been conducting *Voyage to Wellness* cruises throughout the world aboard major cruiselines.

Dr. Taub's one week seminar program aboard ship is designed to allow individuals to experience all the benefits of their cruise vacation, and at the same time, to develop their own *Personal Wellness Plan*. The program is based upon the principles contained in his book *Prescription For Life*, and is designed to help individuals reduce the effects of stress in their lives, loose weight, overcome disease, increase the resistance of their immune systems, and improve the overall quality of their lives.

Now you can benefit from the knowledge that Dr. Taub shares with others during his *Voyage to Wellness* cruises without leaving home. The AWA has recorded the highlights of Dr. Taub's lectures shared with tens of thousands of people aboard ship. The three hour audiocassette package provides an overview of the information contained in Dr. Taub's book, *Prescription For Life*, and outlines the *Personal Wellness Plan* created for you to implement into your life. The cost of the *Voyage to Wellness Lecture Series* is $29.95.

TO ORDER BY CREDIT CARD, CALL TOLL FREE 24 HOURS A DAY FROM ANYWHERE IN THE UNITED STATES, INCLUDING ALASKA AND HAWAII.

1-800-999-1229 EXT. 463

Please indicate the Item Number and quantity you wish to order. Thank You.

Item No.	Description	Price
A-1	Prescription for Life (Book and Audiocassette)	$29.95
A-2	Stress Relief System (8 Audiocassettes)	$99.95
A-3	The Fitness Option (Book and Videotape)	$49.95
A-4	Voyage to Wellness Lecture Series (2 Audiocassettes)	$29.95

AUDIOCASSETTES

A-5	Backache	$11.95
A-6	Weight Loss	$11.95
A-7	Insomnia	$11.95
A-8	Cancer	$11.95
A-9	Alcohol, Smoking and Drug Abuse	$11.95
A-10	Health Rejuvenation	$11.95
A-11	Childhood Illnesses (for parents & children)	$11.95

Chapter One

The Dilemma of the Sick and Tired

TENDER LOVING CARE

Prescription For Life is about healing. As Medicine has become more and more specialized we forgot that such things as a mother's kiss "to make it better" really do help when we are hurting. This book is about tender, loving care that really keeps us well.

So many of us today are hurting, and we don't know who to turn to for our *T.L.C.* Our antacids and surgery, tranquilizers, aspirin and doctors treat only our symptoms, but the real cause of our many discomforts and illnesses won't go away. We are a nation of what I call the "Walking Wounded" and the "Worried Well." The stress we live with is making us age prematurely and experience sickness and dis-ease. For all the technological advances of modern medicine, we are the most over-medicated, over-radiated, operated-upon people in the world. But we are not well!

When patients use the program I present in this book they generally become more healthy and more well than they can possibly imagine.

Prescription For Life is about healing. This is not something anyone else can do for you, but what nature's own healing force — the force that gives us life and works in each of the trillions of cells

1

of our bodies — can do for you if you recognize it, unblock and tap into it, and believe in the power it gives us to control our own health destiny.

The power to heal ourselves, resides in every human cell. It is as awesome and powerful as the force that makes an oak from an acorn. This healing power is evidence of nature's majesty. For the spiritually inclined this power is no less than God's presence in each of our cells. This power makes it absolutely possible, given genetic limitations and some biological constraints, to heal ourselves.

What can unleash our self-healing power? Daily doses of self-administered TLC! And it takes only five weeks to learn how to do this! In just five weeks you will cross a bridge from today's sick and tired feelings to health and aliveness, and the vibrant *Wellness* that ensues will make you God's or Nature's most perfect, most healthy and most admiring fan.

You will learn how all matter — including our bodies, minds, and the neurological pathways on which our thoughts exist — is apparently nothing more than energy. This energy that makes up our thoughts has had a curious history. We are the product of that history and are still creating it today. Our thoughts, as a species, have brought us to our current state of health and dis-ease.

In the beginning (to borrow a well known phrase) the thoughts that first emanated from man's mind allowed him to harness resources to survive: fire, water, grain. Then to domesticate animals, to invent the wheel, to build shelter. Other thoughts led to tribalism and family bonding.

As thoughts gained force and became more comprehensive and systematized, the Stone Age, the Iron Age, and the Bronze Age developed along with more complexity in social systems. And all the while, through all the millennia, thoughts led to more and more sophistication in fulfilling a compelling and all-pervasive historical and instinctual need — to glorify God.

Man began to worship his perceived source of creation. He did so in cave paintings, by constructing monoliths, through chanting and song, by fashioning instruments for music and by building huts, shrines and shelters to house and revere his spiritual *thoughts*—the energy patterns that emanated from his evolving mind.

But occasionally man's thoughts became dark, devious and destructive. To keep the species from extinction, great shifts in consciousness occurred. Certain charismatic individuals appeared to introduce new thoughts and belief systems to the world. These individuals had a sense of sacredness that affected man's thoughts in powerful and long-lasting ways.

Moses appeared with a *law* testament; commandments clearly necessary for survival of a spiritually motivated, but lawless and primitive band of nomads wandering in the Mediterranean basin. This *law* was the basis for what became the Judeo-Christian world view – a prescription for survival.

In Nazareth, Jesus appeared with a testament

of *love*. It was an exact prescription for man kind's thoughts which had recently led to subjugation, slavery and a cruelty that included throwing each other to the lions for sport.

In other parts of the world, enlightened individuals were developing clarity of vision through meditation that focused on wisdom and compassion: Krishna, Buddah, and other individuals all over the earth began reminding people that *thought was only thought and not reality.* Advice and instruction were given that could lead devotees down the paths to nirvana, enlightenment, transcendence of the illusion of their thoughts and to pure bliss. Quite a different path from the one people had begun to walk on, which was leading to disruption, disharmony, discord and death.

But throughout man's history, thoughts period- ically were manipulated in destructive ways in the hands of theologians, kings, queens, emperors, presidents, legislators, physicians, politicians, historians, attorneys, writers and philosophers. The modern dis-ease of man began when the *thoughts* of people with power and influence gained strength and became mistaken for reality and truth. People were *warned* to think only the thoughts of the people in power. All other thoughts, including those that came from instincts, or those that led to tran- scendence, connectedness, and a spiritual reverence for life became branded an illusion that was legally made punishable by ostracism, crucifixion burning and torture.

Only about five hundred years ago man's

survival instinct emerged in a renaissance of
cathedral building attesting again to the glory of
God or a Supreme Being. And soon new religious
leaders again began *insisting* that only their
interpretation of God was real. Governments and
legal systems arose that served lawyers and
legislators who *insisted* only their own thoughts
were correct. Historians began to write history as if
what they wrote was *not* just their thoughts, but
absolute *truth*.

What had been spiritual reality to God loving,
peaceful people, became branded as illusion. <u>*The
thoughts of those in power became reality*</u>. Today
<u>we are in a situation where what we think is real</u>,
<u>may in fact, be an illusion</u>. For it is absolutely
impossible to distinguish reality from illusion. By
definition, illusion is perceived as reality by the
person whose illusion it is. Therefore, what we now
think about God, love, peace, and health is just a
reflection of other people's notions and thoughts:
illusions. When you come right down to it, *thought
is not the same as truth*.

How many of us today still follow the lead of
self-appointed experts? Those institutions that are in
power *still* dictate what we are to believe today.
"Accredited" experts still feel that having babies at
home is primitive and dangerous, that accupuncture
is hokum, that massage is useless, that herbal
medicine is foolish, that science and spirituality
don't mix. How many of us feel foolish when our
instincts tell us to not take certain prescribed
medicine, but to rest, exercise, eat fresh foods,

breathe fresh air? How many experts' books have *you* read in the past few years? How many of them urged you to use your own, powerful inner healing force?

Maimonides was the most famous, influential physician of the twelfth century, acclaimed as a scholar, philosopher and spiritual leader. He emphasized the importance of eating whole grains, warning that refining and processing destroyed health-giving qualities. He strongly recommended avoiding meat and dairy and cautioned against eating certain combinations of food together. He advocated daily vigorous exercise as the best way to keep healthy and repel most disease. Maimonides down-played drugs and surgery (which in those days mostly meant drilling into the skull to remove pieces of it, and bloodletting), arguing that *diet, exercise and mental outlook* were the key determinants of health. He related physical ailments to specific emotional imbalances such as anger, sadness and unrelieved mental stress. He valued meditation, stating clearly that meditation helps self-healing through decreasing evil thoughts, sadness and woes.

But Medicine, once natural and predominantly preventative in nature, saw new people rise to power. In the name of what *they* said was "true science," *they heaped their own thoughts* upon existing thoughts to ultimately develop the incredibly complex system we live with today. The focus of medical care became repairing disease after it had already set in. Knowledge about natural prevention measures and healing with herbs, plants, and foods was ridiculed, banished and forgotten. The sun's healing strength, acupuncture, massage, prayer, faith and meditation gave way to the search for cures after disease had begun. Leeching, purging, and the use of poisons began, and up to only a hundred years ago carpenters' saws and barbers' razors hacked off diseased limbs in operating rooms of dismal filth.

Only decades away from the use of leeches we medicate, radiate, cut, and prescribe harsh and destructive chemicals. We transplant hearts and livers and kidneys. We specialize so much that the doctor of one organ can leave the care of every other organ to doctors who specialize in those organs alone. We perform feats of surgical derring-do putting baboon hearts in human infants. And what does it mean to you? It means that if you are sick you will be cared for in a way that is technologically superb. Yet even as technology applies its surgeries, chemicals, radiation and internal investigations with the latest in medical machinery, you will not be taught to use your innate healing powers to reverse disease and stay well. You will not be prescribed rest, sunshine and natural foods, but you will continue to be poisoned by the salt, sugar, fat, cholesterol, preservatives and chemicals in your diet while you take more and more medicine and undergo more surgical procedures.

I believe it is time to return to more natural, more preventative methods of health care. The razzle-dazzle of technology has made us lose sight of our own natural energy. Our innate self-healing properties have been largely ignored as we've put our health destiny in the hands of technologically proficient experts. It is time to reassert ourselves as our own best health care authorities.

The Prescription for Life will lead you toward independence while it shows you the natural, simple, self-reinforcing, *old fashioned* methods that worked so well for our ancestors, and enabled them to bring us to the world today.

PSYCHONEUROIMMUNOLOGY AND INTEGRATIVE MEDICINE.

Clinical Scientific Medicine has been solidly impacted in the last twenty-five years with an avalanche of data from the science of Psychoneuroimmunology. *The data clearly demonstrates that the way we feel and think can affect our resistance and immunity*.

The *first* revolution that occurred in Medicine during this century was the discovery of antibiotics and the emergence of the quest to find a "magic bullet" for each and every disease. The *second* revolution occurred with super-high technology for diagnosis and treatment leading to "superspecialization" in Medicine. The *third* revolution of our century ushered in by the science of Psychoneuroimmunology, has led to the unprecedented interest in fitness, nutrition, natural and healthy lifestyle, and self-care.

The *fourth* medical revolution of this century will occur through Integrative Medicine because it offers a system of self-empowerment for self-healing. Integrative Medicine is a synthesis of Western Scientific Medicine, Behavioural Medicine, Osteopathic Medicine, Holistic Medicine, Ayurvedic (Indian) Medicine, Homeopathic Medicine, Chiropractic Medicine and Oriental Medicine—*with the addition of a distinctly spiritual component.*

I view patients as three-fold beings: body, mind and spirit. I know my patients become ill mostly because of stress. Their illnesses begin in their mind or persist in their mind. I understand that *ILL* has become equivalent to "I Lack Love" and I am convinced that the body, the mind and the spirit have the ability to reverse any disease—no matter what we have been taught. I have discovered that in this modern age, *health is determined by personal responsibility, self value and reverence for life.* The Prescription For Life is a healing strategy based on this principle. It is effective.

I started developing Integrative Medicine in 1979 because of a feeling of a deep sense of inadequacy. I wanted to help my patients to really and truly be well—*I wanted to teach the hungry to fish rather than merely supplying them with fish.* I now practice Integrative Medicine proudly.

Some of what I say may not make much sense to you—there is a part of your brain that I now call

"*The Thinker*"—I describe it in this book. Your "*Thinker*" will try to stop you from understanding. If you use this book and its accompanying audio cassette tape you will understand.

Psychoneuroimmunology is the science that explores and explains the mind's direct impact on the body—particularly the brain's effect on the immune system. There have been tens of thousands of scientific experiments, tests, and observations during the last twenty-five years that detail the fascinating ways our bodies respond to how we think and feel.

For instance, there are medical studies of patients with multiple personalities that demonstrate that they can have one personality with hypertension and another personality — in the very same body — without hypertension; or one personality that needs very strong eyeglasses and another personality that sees perfectly without eyeglasses; or one personality that gets hives from a particular food allergy and another personality—in the very same body—that has absolutely no problems with the same food.

A now classic study illustrating the mind and body relationship involved a group of individuals who were shown a documentary on Mother Theresa and were then tested for certain immune factors in their blood to measure the potential change in their resistance to disease and their healing response. The tests revealed significantly elevated levels of resistance and healing factors after viewing the film, *even among those viewers who didn't like the film!* This is an example of *immunoenhancement.*

<u>Positive thoughts, feelings and attitudes stimulate</u>
<u>the immune system.</u>

An experiment that I find most interesting involved administering a tuberculosis skin test every month to a group of people with positive reactions. A positive reaction means that the individuals had been exposed to tuberculosis and had developed antibodies to fight the disease. The antibodies cause a red and swollen skin reaction when a tuberculosis-like solution is injected under the skin.

The tuberculosis-like material causing the red and swollen area on the skin of these positive reactors was always used on the *left* arm while a plain inactive water or saline solution was always used on the *right* arm as a control test.

After several months of injections, *without* telling the participants, the tuberculosis material was switched and injected into the right arm and the reddening and swelling did not occur! *Immuno-suppression* occured because of what their minds thought to be so.

We all know we are healthier when we are happy and inspired. That's now new. What is new is that an actual science called Psychoneuroimmun-ology is demonstrating that the immune system affects the nervous system and the nervous system affects the immune system. Our thoughts and feelings surpress or enhance our resistance to disease.

Psychoneuroimmunology uses big words: Immunoglobulins, Thymosins, B-Cells, Plasma

Cells, Macrophages, Lymphocyte T-cells, Neuro-transmitters, Natural Killer Cells, Enkephalins, etc. The big words don't matter. What matters is that Psychoneuroimmunology shows that our innate healing responses become suppressed when we feel hopelessness or experience despair and that our healing force, called *vis medicatrix naturae* by Hippocrates, is enhanced when we feel hardy, optimistic and hopeful.

DIAGNOSTIC ENTRAPMENT

Sarah Wright, is a patient who is sixty-four years old. Her story is typical of tens of thousands of similar stories. Sarah was just not feeling well three years ago. She was chronically tired and fatigued.

She has since seen over twelve physicians — specialists, consultants of the specialists, and consultants of the consultants of the specialists. Sarah has had four prolonged hospital stays for extensive workups and treatment, including stays at the prestigious Scripps Clinic, Cleveland Clinic, Menninger Clinic and Mayo Clinic.

Sarah has given up untold amounts of blood for tests, collected twenty four hours worth of her stools on six occasions and collected her urine for similar amounts of time on seven different occasions —because of questionable findings.

She has been radiated with X-rays that have been repeated many times: X-rays of her chest (eight times), sinuses (three times), abdomen (three times), spine (three times), gall bladder (two times), kidneys (two times), large intestines with barium enemas (three times), stomach and small intestines with barium swallows (three times), long bones, hips, skull and joints (dozens of times). Radioactive substances have also been introduced into Sarah's body to test her thyroid on three occasions, her bones twice, and her blood six times.

Telescope-like tubes have been stuck *up* Sarah's rectum three times, *down* her esophagus twice, *through* her abdomen once, *up* her vagina innumerable times, *down* her windpipe twice and *up* her urethra three times with no diagnosis being made but with more questions surfacing about more and more questionable findings.

Sarah had begun to think she was allergic to wheat. She had been feeling much better as far as "having more energy" and her fatigue had started to lessen about a year ago when she eliminated wheat from her diet.

Unfortunately, the last upper gastro-intestinal series of X-rays, according to the radiologist, "revealed a small polypoid lesion on the greater curvature of the stomach, the significance of which is not clear." The investigation had been complicated by the fact that some "occult blood" had recently been found in one of six daily stool specimens tested. There also seemed to be a "borderline" reversal of the normal albumin-globulin ratio of her blood.

Sarah's tiredness is now returning. She fears she may have cancer—or a rare form of anemia because her last blood test showed some "suspiciously shaped" red cells. Sarah now worries a lot and is fatigued again. She has no energy.

This is not an unusual story, everyone knows similar cases. The woman's diagnosis? Well, Sarah is in her mid-sixties. She's divorced with an adequate settlement and doesn't work. Sarah lives alone and eats mostly junk food and TV dinners. She drinks perhaps a little too much fairly frequently, She doesn't very often see her only child, or grandson who live in New Zealand; she hasn't dated in years, doesn't exercise, has no church affiliation or any really good friends. What do you think?

I think Sarah's story is a dramatic example of how a smouldering sense of hopelessness and despair can lead to a general breakdown of virtually all of the systems of the body. Sarah's story is also a vivid example of what I call "diagnostic entrapment." As medicine becomes more superspecialized and develops more exquisitely sensitive testing procedures, we find more instances of things not being just right which leads to more testing, more expenses and more worry —enough to make a person sick!

Sarah's story is a clinical model of a major concept that will be introduced in this book. **Ill** has become equivalent to **I Lack Love.**

I find it thrilling that research in Psycho-neuroimmunology is now proving what most of us felt we already knew. It was summed all up quite clearly in the *New York Times Magazine* during 1988 when an eminent team of health experts wrote: "The most significant factor in an individual's ability to remain in good health may be a sense of control over the events of life."

My clinical strategy, my actual *Wellness* treatment program is a *biosocial and psycho-spiritual* approach to understanding health and dealing with disease. It is based on Integrative Medicine. I call it the Prescription For Life.

Integrative Medicine enables patients to become effective partners with their physicians. You are about to learn why it is so increasingly necessary for individuals to take responsibility for enhancing their "*Wellness*" —*the healthful balance of body, mind, and spirit.*

I'm pleased to report that Sarah has now completed the Prescription For Life. She is now happier, healthier and more energetic and alive than she ever imagined she could be. Most of all, Sarah now feels autonomous and independent, instead of "trapped" in a diagnostic tunnel without light at the end.

Chapter Two

The Worried Well and The Walking Wounded

INVITATION TO WELLNESS

A re you tired all the time? Are you stressed out, burned out and out of shape? Do you get headaches from time to time? Backaches? How about colds in the winter? The flu too? What about arthritis, high blood pressure, heart problems, allergies, colitis, ulcers, gout, constipation or diarrhea? Do you take antacids after eating a big meal? Do you go to your doctor when you want to feel better? Do you get x-rays, blood and urine tests, injections and prescriptions? Does all this seem perfectly normal to you?

If you answered yes to any of these questions, you have been accepting an invitation to illness. You can just as easily turn down the invitation to doctors, pills, colds, flu, headaches, backaches, heartburn and run down "I-have-no-energy" days.

The Prescription For Life offers a bridge from the sick and tired feeling you may have to total *Wellness* in just five weeks.

If you are a woman, you live in a male-dominated medical society and you are at risk. Hysterectomies (literally "removal of the *craziness*") far outnumber the removal of the testicles (orchid-ectomy, "removal of the *orchids*"). Childbirth is treated as an illness and almost one out of three babies are born via Caesarean section, as if God had erred in not installing a zipper in your abdomen for the easy delivery of your children. You have been taught to believe that this is the price of bearing children. *It is not!*

Your surgically born children are fed chemicals in preference to breast milk. You are told and believe that milk in the cow is equivalent to milk in the breast. Your children are over-medicated during early childhood and overdosing on television whose message reinforces their reliance on junk "food" and medication and develops their expectation of violence, war and sexual promiscuity. When these children reach kindergarten, (now college preparatory in nature), they are further medicated for their "concentration" problems. You have been taught to believe that this is the price of raising children today. *It is not!*

If you are a senior citizen you are prescribed one drug to counteract the effects of another. You may take as many as five or six drugs at a time. These make you drowsy, depressed, confused, impotent, frigid, congested, dizzy and dry. More medication to fight *those* symptoms makes you unable to sleep, causes rashes, interferes with your urination, robs you of energy, makes you irritable and leaves your body in a confused frenzy. Many senior citizens are *"walking side-affects."* You are taught to believe that this is the price of living to old age. *It is not!*

I am writing this book for all of you who have

accepted as your lot in life chronic or acute pain syndromes such as arthritis, coronary problems, backache, headache, and ulcers. I am writing it for victims of allergies. For executives whose stress-filled lifestyle spells the risk of heart disease, strokes, hypertension, myocardial infarctions, gallstones, hemorrhoids, and the certainty of being out of touch with self and family. You have been taught to accept your condition as inevitable. *It is not!*

As a species we must always experience disease when it is time to die to replenish the species – like the fields of flowers that wilt at the end of spring. But in this age of stress with our destructive habits and lifestyles, our powerful medicines and frequent surgeries, radiation, smog, depleted ozone, acid rain, and continuous exposure to violence, almost all disease is occuring *prematurely.*

My goal is to teach you what *Wellness* is. To show you how to achieve it in five weeks. To show you how the illness-producing thoughts in our society conspire to keep you ill, and how you can recognize them to render them impotent. I will show you how to introduce *Wellness*-producing thoughts to take their place.

I will show how disease results from the *mind's* cooperation with the body. When I say disease depends on the mind's cooperation with the body, I am not "blaming the victim" for his or her disease. A two-year old with leukemia does not bring on the illness. *But* when something is not working right in the *body*, something is not working right in the *mind* as well, for the *mind regulates the body*. In fact, our belief that the mind and body are separate is an illusion. *Every thought we think is instantly transmitted to and reflected in each and every cell in our bodies.* Nothing in the body happens by chance. Everything physical is carefully regulated. *Wiggle your finger in a glass of water and all the water molecules become agitated. Think a thought and every cell in the body feels the effect.*

I will show you how to harness your mind's energy to keep disease out of your life. I will show you how you can even harness your genetic potentials to keep you well. I will offer you a total induction to health and an introduction to Integrative Medicine. I will teach you how you, and you alone, can determine your own degree of *Wellness.*

You can think of this book as a manual for your health care. It is meant to instill an awareness in you. Once that awareness is there, you will automatically begin to become well. Your belief systems, whether you are aware of them or not, are what make you sick or keep you healthy. I invite you to learn how these belief systems work, how to reprogram those that don't serve you well, and install in their place a new awareness that can keep you healthy and feeling terrific.

NEW ENGLAND JOURNAL OF MEDICINE...

- **80% OF DISEASE IS NOT HELPED BY MEDICINE AND SURGERY**

- **10% OF DISEASE IS HELPED BY MEDICINE AND SURGERY**

- **10% OF DISEASE IS *CAUSED* BY MEDICINE AND SURGERY**

Inglefinger, F.J., Health: A Matter of Statistics or Feeling, New England Journal of Medicine, February 24, 1977, 448-449.

The *New England Journal of Medicine* reported in 1977, that *eighty percent of the illness and symptoms of Americans cannot be helped by medicine and surgery at all!* The Journal went on to state that medication and surgery currently help only ten percent of illness and that medicine and surgery actually cause *ten percent of illness.*

And, in 1979 the then Secretary of Health, Education and Welfare, Joseph Califano, and the leading medical authority in the United States, the Surgeon General, Julius Richmond, M.D., declared, *"The health of the American people in the 1980's will depend on what they are willing to do for themselves, and not on what others are willing to do for them."*

The implications of that declaration carried special weight for me because Doctor Julius Richmond had been my professor and "guiding light" in medical school. Could it be that we doctors were really helping so few? Could it be that the majority of patients really could heal themselves?

In my own practice I began to study the charts, financial ledgers and appointment patterns and I discovered a shocking phenomenon:

Twenty percent of my patients were sick eighty percent of the time!

Twenty percent of my practice was utilizing eighty percent of my professional time and was responsible for eighty percent of my office visits and income! Conversely, the other eighty percent of my patients were sick and coming in to see me only twenty percent of the time.

I fought to resist what I was seeing because the enormous personal and professional significance of the phenomenon was immediately evident. It could alter my entire view of illness and disease, and change the way I had been taught to practice Medicine.

I fully expected that the families and kids who were sick most of the time would be the leukemics or cases of juvenile rheumatoid arthritis, or inherited immune deficiencies or genetic syndromes. But they were not! The twenty percent of the patients who were sick eighty percent of the time were those who were merely experiencing troublesome but nonspecific illness and disease, including:

1. **Aches and Pains:** migraine, arthralgia, lumbosacral spasm, arm and leg discomfort, swellings.
2. **Upper Respiratory Problems:** congestion, allergy, fullness, dripping, coughing, sneezing.
3. **Gastrointestinal Problems:** constipation, diarrhea, eating too much, eating too little, gas, bloating, colitis, ileitis, proctitis, bleeding hemorrhoids, ulcers.

4. **Skin Problems:** rashes, eczema, psoriasis, itching, scratching, redness, paleness, dryness.
5. **Learning and Behavioral Difficulties:** dyslexia, hyperactivity, neurosis, anorexia, phobias, truancy, vandalism, alcohol, drugs.
6. **Repeat Infections:** otitis, tonsillitis, bronchitis, gastroenteritis, sinusitis, cystitis, pyelonephritis.

I am a traditionally seasoned clinician. I attended an excellent school and had superb specialty training. I'm skilled at diagnosis and treatment. But I could not find any defect or deficiency to explain the compilation of human misery just detailed. It was *just happening*, and people and families accepted it and *thought* it perfectly normal to visit the doctor's office several times a year. They *thought* it perfectly normal to raise kids with recurring abdominal pains, rashes, multiple episodes of ear infections and tonsillitis, or repeated coughs, colds and runny noses.

The conclusion was inescapable. Patients who were sick most of the time had no discernible reason for illness, no genetically predetermined syndromes or specific disease entities. These patients were what I came to call the "Worried Well" and the "Walking Wounded."

Children and adults had become so used to illness that they had lost sight of the light at the end of the tunnel. They relied on their doctor to be a *pill fairy*.

These patients or their families carried a conviction — a thought — with them: *that illness*

was a natural, expected and frequent part of life.
They expected illness, anticipated sickness, were
convinced of its regular occurrence, and adapted a
"wait for it" attitude.

On the other hand, the eighty percent of families
who hardly ever utilized my services other than for
regularly scheduled checkups were *qualitatively*
different from the "Worried Well" and the
"Walking Wounded." The difference had no
relationship to socioeconomic factors or to race.
Their healthiness was clearly associated with an
attitude.

The well families had a major, common
characteristic. Their attitude was one of *not having
time to be sick, not expecting to be sick, and not
wanting to have anything to do with being sick.*
Illness was far removed from their expectation and
everyday thought. The very notion of becoming sick
appeared to be a vague and distant concept to these
patients and their families who seemed happier,
more optimistic and carefree. They appeared not
very stressed or worried. The differences between
the two groups were obvious even in tiny infants
who were more playful and relaxed in the well
group, responding to my examining hands with
laughter and delight as their parents looked on,
comfortable and relaxed.

As I spent more time evaluating the frame of
mind and the attitude of these patients, the meaning
of *Wellness* began to make sense to me.

WHAT WELLNESS IS!

Wellness is difficult to describe to people who have never experienced it. It is so much more than just an absence of symptoms that unless you have known its effect it is hard to believe it really exists.

Wellness is a physical, emotional and spiritual state of health that manifests itself through joyful, energetic living. Not only does *Wellness* truly exist, it is easily within anyone's grasp! It is not only for those who are lucky, those with good genes. It is for *you* even if you now take medication, don't sleep well at night, don't have as much energy as you would like or don't feel as well as you would like. *Wellness* can be yours in five weeks even if you are anxious, hypertensive, depressed, grieving, lonely, overweight, diabetic or in any way "*sick and tired.*"

The Prescription For Life can work for you if you are really ready to be well. If you truly believe you want to be well, you can be. The belief element is absolutely crucial to this program.[1]

---

[1] Herbert Benson's book, BEYOND THE RELAXATION RESPONSE (Morrow, 1975), talks about the belief element in meditation and prayer and its physiological effect in stress reduction.

ILLNESS INDUCING THOUGHTS

Tens of millions of Americans are part of the "Walking Wounded" and "Worried Well." Our minds are programmed to be ill almost from the moment we are born (and some would say before). Sickness-inducing thoughts are constantly being infused into our brains through television, radio, newspapers, magazines, movies, songs, books, advertisements and through the usually well-intentioned efforts of doctors, hospitals, charities for disease, schools, parents and friends. If this is a new concept to you, let me give you a few examples.

Every time you see an ad on TV for Tums, Anacin, Dristan, Contact, Excedrin, Preparation H, or DiGel, *disease is brought to mind and the idea is reinforced that it is time to have: an upset stomach, stuffed nose, achy flu, headaches, hemmorhoids, or acid indigestion.* On a subtle level your mind accepts these hundreds of billions of dollars of advertisments and registers that the next time you have any of these symptoms, there is a solution available, an end to your discomfort that you can buy.

Remember that each thought you have is instantaneously reflected in every cell in your body (just like all the molecules were in a glass of water that you wiggled your finger in). Can you see how these messages are illness-inducing thoughts to buy the economy size, double strength brand "X"

Medicine?

When you read the newspaper and some doctor predicts that some specific number of people will come down with some specific disease within the next year, your mind registers that perhaps you will be among those he is dooming to ill health. Can you see how this is an illness-inducing thought?

When *USA TODAY* quotes (as it did on February 20, 1986) a high ranking official of the American Academy of Pediatrics suggesting, *It is normal and expected that your child will be ill for twenty to thirty days a year until two or three years old,* your mind registers that it is expected that your child visits the doctor frequently. After all, if a high ranking pediatrician says it is normal for baby to be ill *ten percent of the time,* who are you to argue? Can you see how this is an illness-inducing thought? You are constantly being conditioned to think this way!

When the mother of a small child says, "Don't go outside with wet hair; you'll catch a cold!" or "Walking around without shoes will make you sick," or "Don't get caught in the rain; you'll catch pneumonia," or any other such warning, that child also registers the message and carries it for life. Can you see how this (even though the mother's intentions are loving) is an illness-inducing thought?

When something is predicted, or just constantly "*brought to mind*" it stimulates the potential in your mind for it to occur. In fact, often the stress resulting from the prediction is the key that unlocks the disease that was predicted. How often have doctors, in announcing how long a patient has to live, sentenced that patient to death?

The media are an especially dangerous predictor and cause of disease. A clear example of the media's negative influence on our health can be seen with anorexia, bulemia and other eating disorders. Newspaper articles, magazines, novels, movies, songs and advertisements, are actually causing diseases for which we then have to create an entire industry. We are starting to witness such a phenomenon with teenage suicide, Temporal Mandibular Joint Dysfunction, Premenstrual Syndrome, Ebstein-Barr Virus, Mitral Valve Prolapse, Chronic Pain Sydrome, and Osteoporosis.

Let me explain. I was a board certified pediatrician and medical school teacher for almost fifteen years with an established reputation as a specialist in Adolescent Medicine. During all my time in practice, and with roughly twenty thousand patients my clinic cared for, I came across only *three* children with the eating disorders anorexia nervosa and bulimia. Two cases were barely eating at all, the other eating well, but making herself vomit. All three cases had deeply suppressed sexual fantasies. They were teen-aged girls (the disease had hardly ever been known to occur otherwise).

My three cases in fifteen years made me somewhat of a local specialist in eating disorders. I lectured at "Grand Rounds" at the medical school; authors, mostly budding young psychologists interviewed me for their scholarly papers. Now, ten years later, we have created a disease that has

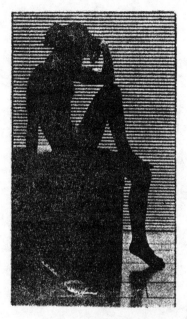

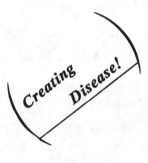

Creating Disease!

ARE YOU LOSING IT?

"I'm lonely and confused. Not eating is my choice."
"My child is starving herself and I'm frightened."
"I binge to make myself happier and then force myself to throw up. It makes me feel better for awhile . . . a little while."

These are thoughts and feelings expressed by people whose lives are affected by serious eating disorders.

Losing sight of yourself . . . your feelings . . . your eating habits can be dangerous. **Anorexia Nervosa, Bulimia** and **Compulsive Overeating** are eating disorders often resulting from deep hurt and pain.

At ⬛⬛⬛ Hospital, we understand the loneliness and confusion you are feeling. All of us working with the Eating Disorders Program are here to help and listen. You *can* get better. And we have the specialists who can show you how. Unlike many other programs, ⬛⬛⬛ Hospital does not group you with patients suffering from obesity or various addictive illnesses.

Call us any time of the day or night for confidential help. Consultation is free throughout your decision-making process.

"My sister is starving herself to death."

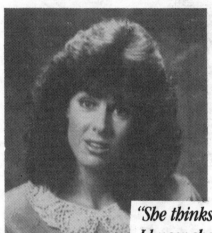

"She thinks she's fat, but I know she is too thin. Much too thin. I'm worried... she says she's too busy to eat, but I'm afraid it's more than that. She's obsessed with her weight. What could be wrong with her?"

24 Hour Hotline

Treatment Center

become rampant. The media has created *eating disorders* as a common and expected option for teenagers. They see it in first-run movies, read about it in best-selling novels, and watch it on heartbreaking television shows. Newspapers and magazines have been reporting that up to *ten percent* of all teenage girls are afflicted and, indeed, now the media reports that boys are getting it, too. *And they are!*

Advertisements for specialized anorexia and bulimia hospital care units, residential treatment centers, even resorts, fill the health pages of newspapers. Bold headlines offer help for the eating disorder epidemic! This epidemic has been created in the mind! The expectancy and anticipation of anorexia and bulimia in the teenage population has got kids fasting and vomiting away in droves! And this new problem is being fueled by a newly budding industry of super-specialists who care for *eating disorders*. It is reminiscent of the middle ages when as many people purportedly died from fright of the plague bacillus as did from actual infection.

Teenage suicides are similarly being fueled by the media. Kids get the idea it is expected that suicides occur in waves and in groups. They feel themselves at risk and thoughts begin to attack them when a schoolmate commits suicide. They *"know"* that three or four schoolmates are supposed to do the same thing. Parents *"know"* too. I am not asking that the news media not report on what is happening. But what is dangerous is that "experts" are called on to predict what *will* happen, and these often become self-fulfilling prophecies. It is one thing to report that a teenager committed suicide. It is quite another thing – a more dangerous thing – to extrapolate from that incident what *number* of teenagers are likely contemplating suicide and how many are *expected* to occur. The prediction makes teenagers worry that maybe they will be the next statistic. And now a teenager commits suicide almost every thirty minutes in the United States! *The suicide option is real and its persistant image really does induce stress.*

Just as a doctor's prediction of how long a patient will live affects the quality and length of that patient's survival, so report after report and expert after expert predicting how many people will develop an eating disorder syndrome, or attempt suicide, or have allergies, or develop a breast lump, will affect the outcome of those predictions.

Until four or five years ago, Osteoporosis was a condition that was basically familiar to every doctor, but really no big deal. Only a rather expected consequence of aging, and usually found in women. It was usually found quite incidentally, recognized on routine chest x-rays without much thought being given to it at all. (If your doctor is over 35, he will remember this. Ask him!) We knew about Osteoporosis and occasionally suggested calcium if we found the condition, but we rarely looked for it or attempted to diagnose it as a specific disease process causing any specific symptoms. Now, thanks to the media, the milk industry, the vitamin manufacturers and the invention of expensive high-tech machinery to screen for the condition, Osteoporosis has become a leader of *national hype!* Everything from poor posture to dying like a withered old pretzel is being beaten into our imaginations as tens of millions of scared women go for Osteoporosis screenings, buy more milk, swallow more expensive minerals and support this new industry!

The specter of disease can trigger the disease— particularly under stress! And in our stressed-out society, almost all illness begins in the mind. Advertising on TV, radio and in newspapers and magazines can make you feel and experience the discomfort of everything from headaches to diarrhea. Even the lobbying of good-willed people working for the cancer, arthritis, diabetes, or M.S. foundations, trying to bring specific illnesses to your attention, contributes to your constant exposure to illness inducing thoughts. Keep this in mind as you look at magazines or watch TV from now on. One recent ad showed a woman saying, "I thought I had a bad cold. Then I found out it was asthma. *Was I glad*!" She was glad, presumably, because there is an industry that can 'help' the woman with her asthma –for a price, to be sure. She can visit the specialist who ran the ad—what a relief! She has a chronic condition complete with its own experts instead of a virus that would go away on its own!

Another recent ad warned that spring is just around the corner. It suggested that you visit your allergy specialist *before* you notice your first

The first symptom in 40% of all heart attacks is
SUDDEN DEATH

The really sad part is that it doesn't have to be that way. For just one hour of your time and $105, you can find out what your chances are of having a heart attack.

As a community service, along with the fine hospitals listed below, will co-sponsor Cardiac Risk Factor Identification Programs during the next few weeks. Each individual participating in this program will receive a Resting EKG, an Exercise Stress EKG, a Pulmonary Function Test, Blood Chemistry tests (including cholesterol, HDL level, triglyceride level, and fasting blood sugar), and percent body fat analysis.

To participate in any of the one day programs listed please call

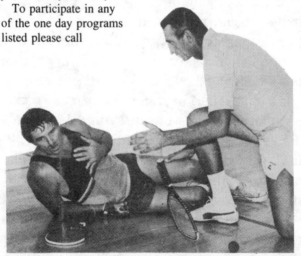

Doesn't this cause you mental Stress?
Your body is responding too!

IS BREAST CANCER
IN YOUR FUTURE?

NOW IT IS ALMOST IMPOSSIBLE FOR BREAST CANCER TO REMAIN HIDDEN. At WOMAN AWARE Diagnostic Center, a Woman's Medical Center, the world's finest and newest diagnostic equipment is used to find malignancies long before they can be felt. With one in 10 women now destined to get breast cancer, it is increasingly imperative to find it early. With early diagnosis over 90% of breast malignancies can be removed without extensive surgery.

At 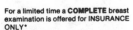 we use new low-dose xeromammography instead of the older film screen X-ray as it will visualize the breast all the way to the rib cage where ordinary film screen X-ray mammography does not and cannot reach. Also, abnormalities are much more easily seen with the images from our equipment.

Because almost all women between the ages of 35-50 have both dense and fatty tissue in their breasts, and mammography does not visualize thru dense tissue, Dedicated ultrasound scanning is recommended to obtain the maximum visualization. The combination of these two modalities increases the diagnostic capability of mammography to as high as 98%. Mammography alone is less than 70% diagnostic.

For a limited time a **COMPLETE** breast examination is offered for INSURANCE ONLY*

* Low-dose Xeromammography
* Computerized Ultrasound Scan— **(NO RADIATION)** includes complete video and film record for future comparison
* Breast examination and training in self-examination
* Physician consult
* Radiologist report
* Pleasant and supportive surroundings

A visit to will give you the peace of mind that only the best examination obtainable can give you.

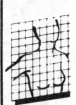

Doesn't this stress your mind?
It does the same to your body!

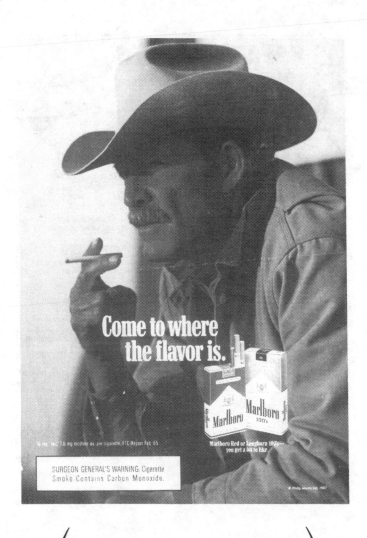

Come to where
the flavor is.

SURGEON GENERAL'S WARNING: Cigarette
Smoke Contains Carbon Monoxide.

Marlboro Red or Longhorn 100's—
you get a lot to like.

$$\left(\begin{array}{c}\textit{Mental Programming:}\\ \textit{"Cigarettes are for REAL men"}\end{array}\right)$$

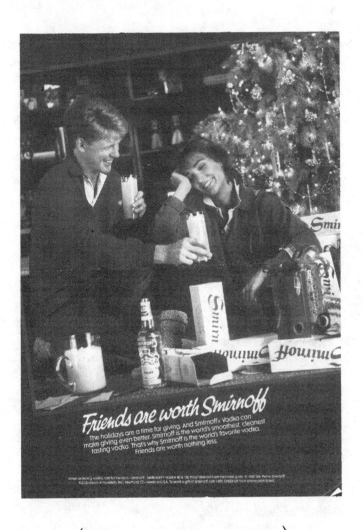

Friends are worth *Smirnoff*

The holidays are a time for giving. And Smirnoff Vodka can make giving even better. Smirnoff is the world's smoothest, cleanest tasting vodka. That's why Smirnoff is the world's favorite vodka. Friends are worth nothing less.

$$\left(\begin{array}{c}\textbf{\textit{Mental Programming:}}\\ \textbf{\textit{``Alcohol helps friendship''}}\end{array}\right)$$

symptoms! These advertisers would have you equate an entire season of every year with illness!

Could this be a significant factor in the onset of cancer too? What about the predicition that 100% of people with positive AIDS tests will die of the disease. What could this do?

Worry depresses minds that have already been so heavily programmed. You have been receiving these illness-supporting messages for so long, subconsciously accepting them for so long, that it is difficult to suddenly recognize them for what they are. The Prescription For Life helps you open your mind to examine the swarming mass of thoughts programmed into it that are inviting you to illness. Once you see that your mind is locked into a powerful program of illness-inducing attitudes and thoughts, you will be able to choose *Wellness* or illness. You will make an *informed* choice, not feel victimized.

SICK BUSINESS

Americans are getting sick to the tune of *five hundred billion dollars a year*. We are manu-facturing enough tranquilizers for every man, woman and child in the country to have one a day. If *you* are not taking one a day, *someone else* is taking your share! We produce enough aspirin for every man, woman, child and infant to take two hundred and eighty a year! If you are not taking yours, then again someone has gotten your share. *Now it is getting worse as the advertising image is being created in your mind that somehow you may have a heart attack if you are "aspirin deficient."*

Once you understand how illness or *Wellness* is your own choice, often you will see that by choosing illness you are doing what is *expected* of you by our country. Does this seem absurd to you? Consider the following. . . Twelve percent of our gross national product is spent to repair disease (compared to less than one tenth of one percent to promote *Wellness*). Hospitals, doctors, drug companies, ambulances, insurance, x-ray companies, vitamin manufacturers, advertising agencies, surgical suppliers, charity leagues, the stock market and tens of millions of people in the work force *are depending on you to be sick!*

Even natural processes like birth and death are treated as sickness. In many areas of the country being born costs one thousand dollars a day! Almost one in three births is by caesarean section. And dying, now to be avoided at any cost, finally does cost tens of thousands of dollars in hospital fees, sometimes with as many as four or five cardiopulmonary resuscitations before you're permitted to breathe your last breath.

Actually, about five hundred billion dollars a year, *another* twelve percent of our economy is spent on *getting* you sick in the first place! The alcohol, tobacco and junk food industry and all the companies that pollute the air are doing just that — getting you sick.

By *not* being well and by *expecting* doctors and hospitals, nose sprays, aspirin and stomach pills to repair you when you are ailing, you are supporting big business! Medicine has traditionally concentrated on disease repair. Surgery and drugs treat the symptoms and not the causes of disease; they do not "heal," but fix. *Wellness* counts on your own, natural self-healing abilities. If you are truly well, you do not need the big businesses that count on you to remain sick and tired! When you are truly well, many businesses and professionals will go out of business. In fact, today many forward-looking segments of the healing professions *are* starting to do just that: get out of the old disease repair business and into the new, real health care, the business of staying well.

Wellness is the most powerful and concentrated healing state the body can be in. It has the potential to reverse any disease if the tissue or cellular structure is still alive. *Wellness* encompasses a view of your world as nurturing, friendly and being there to support you in health.

MIRACLE HEALINGS

There are millions of documented examples of remarkable recoveries from illness and remarkable survivals from near death that traditional scientists have labelled miraculous. In fact these are miraculous, but they are not mysterious. They are miraculous because our human life is a miracle! Traditional Medicine and traditional science count on laboratory results to confirm their findings. Under the current system, any theory or treatment of disease is not accepted until it has been "proven" by a number of repetitions. Adequate data and scientific measurement are required. This ability to duplicate the results of a diagnostic and therapeutic procedure is the scientific basis of the current disease repair medical system, but it is also one of its major pitfalls, since *any healing that doesn't fit the pattern is apt to be discarded as a fluke, an aberration.* If someone feels better, regains health, sends his disease into remission, modern Medicine cannot account for the changes if one of its practitioners or procedures wasn't included in the therapy. Even the language of modern Medicine reflects the doctor's belief that the patient has little or nothing to do with his or her own health and healing. "The cancer went into remission," (which is often as close as a doctor will ever come to saying, "we don't know why the disease went away"), is typical of the way doctors make the disease the subject of the sentence. The disease itself is given power to come and go with no acknowledgement of the patient's role. But where laboratories and traditional science tend to be lacking is one the human, spiritual side of healing.

Every year, tens of thousands of people experience what we physicians call "idiopathic spontaneous remissions." "Idiopathic spontaneous remission" is what we call it when a serious, often catastrophic dis-ease just goes away and we don't know why.

I have asked hundreds of patients with "idiopathic spontaneous remissions" involving serious diseases

what happened. Almost all of them say: *"I just
didn't have time for it,"* — *"I wasn't going to be
bothered by it,"* — *I just wasn't going to to let it get
me,"* or *"I just prayed and put myself totally in
God's hands!"*

In any case, your attitude, particularly your
level of "hardiness" — that's your optimism and
mental strength is a crucial factor that stimulates
your healing powers and assists your physician to
help you.

People who feel good about themselves, about
the world and about others, — *who believe in a
higher power or a supreme being* — are generally
much more happy and well than people who are
pessimistic, depressed, angry and feeling hopeless.

Wellness encompasses the human, spiritual
side of life to explain and harness the life energy that
causes these "miraculous" healings that medical
science cannot explain. Integrative Medicine understands that body, mind and spirit work best when
they are recognized as different forms of the same
energy.

Just as ice, water and steam are different forms
of H_2O, so your life energy is your life energy
whether you are talking about your body, your
mind, or your spirit. Thoughts don't exist only in
your mind. Every thought you have is transmitted
by a complex pathway to every cell in your body.
On a cellular level your body responds to everything
you see, smell, hear, or imagine. Your body – *every
cell in your body* – responds to every violent scene
you witness in a movie or in the street. On a cellular

level your body *responds* to every TV commercial you see (including those that bring illness to mind in order for you to use certain products to stop your symptoms). Every time you have an argument, every time someone criticizes you, offers you a diagnosis, or engages your mind in any way, your *entire* body responds. Imagine how differently your body would respond to these messages if the messages were peaceful and not violent; if the TV sold prevention and not repair.

THOUGHT ENERGY

Imagine that your life energy flows from your mind to your body and from your body to your mind.

When a river is flowing freely it is very powerful. Anyone who has seen the Grand Canyon knows that the force of the Colorado River carved a sculpture so large and so beautiful it inspires awe. When the energy of your mind and body are allowed to flow freely, when the blocks that are damming the flow are understood and let go, you will experience with new awe the absence of fatigue, the absence of illness and its symptoms, the absence of that sick and tired feeling and a powerful, joyful energy that is no less magnificent than the Grand Canyon itself!

According to your choice and your will, your mind can be a raging river or a calm ocean. Neither the river or the ocean is good or bad, neither is right or wrong. Nature creates both, and both are powerful forces. The secret I want to share with you is that you have the ability to control that mighty force. You use it now without knowing it, and it is that powerful force *misdirected or blocked* that is making you feel less than 100 percent. Once you learn how *Wellness*, just like illness, begins in your mind; once you understand that your thoughts are powerful and your beliefs are powerful, you will be more able to harness that power and consciously choose illness or *Wellness*, fatigue or energy. The choice can be yours! You can be the master of your health destiny.

You have been building dams that stop the flow or redirect the natural flow of your personal, powerful, *Wellness*-directed energy. What you learn can enable you to stop building these barriers (made of junk "food," salt, sugar, tobacco, drugs, alcohol, pollution, smog, radiation, media advertisements for illness, even unnecessary surgery).

Let's put all this into perspective. It should now be clearer to you how important your own responsibility is for your health — just as the Surgeon General of the United States so effectively stated. And, if 80% of your disease cannot be helped by others, it should be clear how much you must do for yourself. The necessity of your assuming a partnership with your doctor should be evident. Your healing power is greater than anything that exists in your doctor's black bag or in the halls of the Mayo Clinic. Understanding this, you can begin an effective partnership for life.

Let me explain to you now how Integrative

Medicine differs from *Traditional* Medicine, and how it can help you cross the bridge from sick and tired to healthy and well.

Chapter Three

The Endangered Mind

REVERENCE FOR LIFE

I ntegrative Medicine enables you to be well and stay well. It does not encourage return trips to the doctor. It does not encourage you to take medication if natural alternatives can work as well. Integrative Medicine is called that because it promotes the concept of integrity of body, mind and soul for the individual. It offers the integration of technology and intuition for the medical doctor who has come to rely on technology alone. Integrative Medicine promotes your *Wellness*, not your illness. It teaches prevention, not repair.

Integrative Medicine is a cooperative process that uses the patient's own healing resources. You cannot be as well with anybody else's help as you can be if your own healing powers are brought into play. Integrative Medicine gives the patient the power and responsibility to heal and be healthy.

In my practice alone, Integrative Medicine has reached tens of thousands of people from age four to eighty-six. You will meet some of them in these pages.

A basic understanding of Integrative Medicine is that faith, *just a willingness to believe,* can bring about miracles in disease reversals. Everyone knows someone who has gotten well against all odds. Some people call it a "will to live." As I have previously said, physicians refer to unexplained and sometimes dramatic disease reversals as spontaneous idiopathic remissions. It means that they don't know what happened! Today, Medicine tends to push these cases aside while it continues to look only for statistical validation. Remissions like these are treated as flukes. But these are important data and we can no longer ignore them!

In practice, Integrative Medicine is non-judgmental about the tools of healing. It puts at the mind's and body's disposal *all* healing possibilities, not just those we have used in Western Medicine during the twentieth century (which is what you have typically experienced until now in conventional office settings or hospitals). Whereas "modern" Medicine is unable to measure the quality of healing in any terms but the technological (which, unfortunately often ends up treating the patient as a piece of machinery), Integrative Medicine allows the patient to measure "How are you?" in very human terms.

In an Integrative Medicine practice you will find any kind of help, ranging from a CAT scan to a consultation with a minister or nutritionist, or a discussion of ancient healing methods. I use penicillin and surgery as well as accupuncture and healing herbs, massage and spinal adjustment as well as physical therapy; and most importantly, meditation, faith and prayer. The key point is *primum non nocere,* first do no harm. Then

I choose the most natural, least expensive and least harmful therapy that addresses the cause of the patient's disease instead of just its symptoms. This book is about "Abettors" of Wellness and will inroduce you to the wide range of healing possibilities you can use with or without the help of others.

"Abettors" of *Wellness* — Primary Factors

Fresh Air, Sunshine & Rest
Fresh Fruit
Fresh Vegetables
Raw Nuts
Whole Grains
Friends
Pets
Hobbies
Service to Others
Honesty
Massage
Yoga
Safety
Meditation and Prayer
Gardening
Laughing, Singing, Playing
Loving
Walking, Jogging, Aerobics
Swimming, Tennis, Golf, Skiing, Team Sports

Secondary Factors

Innoculation
Medicine
Surgery
Radiation

Unlike Integrative Medicine, our present illness-oriented medical system concentrates almost entirely on detecting and describing disease and abolishing signs and symptoms through medication, surgery, radiation and psychotherapy. It also formulates public health laws and immunizes patients against contagious disease. In fact, modern (Western) Medicine as we know it has tremendous validity. Until the recent epidemic of new sexually transmitted disease, it had lifted almost entirely the burden of *infectious* disease (smallpox, typhus, diphtheria, polio, tuberculosis for example) from industrialized society in this century alone. But it has not dealt well with the *degenerative* diseases that are modern society's plague (heart disease, hypertension, diabetes, arthritis, respiratory problems, and cancer are the most prevalent of these). Modern Medicine has only just begun to look at all disease in the larger context of stress, the environment, and the patient's values and belief system.

Integrative Medicine has been developing as an effort from *within* the medical system, to accelerate this broader outlook. If Medicine until now is a hospital that has served us very well, but is overcrowded and in need of renovation, Integrative Medicine provides the new space that will allow room for new thoughts about old procedures. It will also eliminate the need for overcrowded hospitals as people learn how they are responsible for their own health. According to Integrative Medicine,

health is determined by personal responsibility, self-value, and reverence for life.

A LITTLE HISTORY AND A LOT OF TECHNOLOGY

Medicine, as taught and practiced today in the United States, is an extraordinary system based on discoveries, theories, and inventions that, for the most part, surfaced during the last hundred years: Louis Pasteur's work with microbes, Robert Koch's postulates on infectious disease, Paul Ehrlich's discovery that he could create a magic cure called Sulfa, and Selman Waxman's and Alexander Fleming's observation that nature itself was creating Streptomycin and Penicillin.

Within this century a chemical revolution was born, and the predominant thrust in medicine became finding or inventing a *silver bullet* to repair any disease.

The effort to prevent, reverse or cure through *better chemicals* changed the context of medical training. What had been a somewhat ragtag system of nostrums, notions and tonics dispensed by anyone from distinguished physicians to local "barber-surgeons," became a licensed course of study.

This new field of medical study developed tools

to enlarge its scope: stethoscope, otoscope (used to view the middle ear), ophthalmoscope (used to see the retina), sigmoidoscope (used to examine the rectum and colon), oscilloscope (a screen that shows electrical waves), microscope, all the way to present-day electron and ultra-electron microscope. New training curricula developed to justify, codify, explain and make sense of everything being found through all the new *scopes* of exploration.

The training of physicians and surgeons began to include the study of histology (tissue structure), anatomy, biochemistry, microbiology and physiology. The thrust of medical work became detection, labelling and describing disease, abolishing symptoms and making the patient feel more comfortable as quickly as possible.

Something got lost in all this. Medical training today does not include a strong vision of internal turmoil, stress and unhealthy lifesytles as important to the onset of disease. Very little time is spent to make doctors aware of how important personal choices are in determining illness or health, degeneration or healing. In the standard texts of general learning used by most medical schools today (Cecil, Loeb, and Harrison's textbooks of Internal Medicine), there are tens of thousands of subjects in the index, but *"healing"* is not listed!

Medicine today may do as much harm as good. As explained earlier, medicine and surgery may only help us ten percent of the time, and now may actually *cause* ten percent of our illness. Eighty percent of all ailments may not be helped by medicine or surgery at all. Yet trying to eliminate headaches, aspirin has become as common in millions of households as a prayer before a meal used to be. Trying to deal with stress, tranquilizers have become a way of life for millions of Americans. It was the famous former Justice Oliver Wendell Holmes who said that if you took the entire American pharmacoepia – all the drugs available – and tossed it in the ocean, it would be so much better for man, *and so much worse for the fish!*

Doctors today spend very little time helping you understand why you got sick in the first place. The doctor may tell his diabetic patient to eat less, or the smoker to stop smoking or the alcoholic to quit drinking or the anxious patient to "loosen up." But other than facts and fear (telling the diabetic he may lose a leg or the smoker a lung) or medication (tranquilizers for the anxiety-ridden), the doctor in many instances does not have skills to influence patients to change. *Facts and fear are very poor motivators of healthful change.* (People continue to smoke and refuse to wear seat belts.) Even many doctors have not yet adopted their own advice concerning health and continue to overeat and lead stressful lives. *Optimal health care, whatever your need is, can only be achieved when you as a patient assume your crucial role with your physician in a partnership for your own life.*

BEGINNINGS OF INTEGRATIVE MEDICINE

Integrative Medicine emphasizes that stress is the major cause of the diseases we experience: the migraines, backaches, ulcers, colds, heart attacks, strokes, and even arthritis and cancer in very many instances. (The theory of templates introduced in chapter four will help you understand this).

Stress has become an overwhelming problem today for two major reasons:

1. Modern medical practice is not equipped to handle stress; very little is taught to medical students about dealing with fear, anxiety, economic insecurity, grief or loneliness.

2. The greatest cause of stress is our thoughts and the way we think. *Stress begins between our ears*! Unless we can tap into our thought processes in a healthful way, stress and its effects become a vicious cycle.

Medical students don't learn effective ways to treat stress. They learn to tranquilize, institutionalize, electroshock and refer to psychiatrists, whose practices Ashley Montague described as "the study of the id by the odd." (This may sound flippant, but if a shaman from somewhere in Central Asia looked at Freud, penis envy and castration complexes, he might well mutter, "What an exotic belief system!")

As a practicing pediatrician, I became painfully aware of the number of stress-related illnesses I was treating. The colic, allergy, sore throats, gastro-

intestinal diseases, coughs, colds, earaches, runny
noses, rashes, failure to thrive and behavioral and
educational disorders were overwhelmingly stress
induced! Many children with frequent colds, ear
infections, bronchitis and tonsillitis were *physically*
stressed by living in a household where one or both
parents smoke; the cilia (hairs) in the child's
respiratory passages, bathed in smoke, were
numbed and could not perform their function of
keeping the passages clear.

Children with asthma were often *emotionally*
stressed from families with high levels of anxiety.
The children frequently seemed to be suppressed in
their abilities to express themselves and say or do
what was on their minds. Many seemed to wheeze
when they needed attention and nurture.

Many children with respiratory problems were
stressed by the loads of milk they were being fed. (I
felt some remorse for the years when I had
snickered with my colleagues at the mothers who
insisted that milk made their children congested and
mucousy. This has now become widely accepted in
connection with respiratory ailments including
allergies. I have learned to listen very carefully to
mothers' observations.)

Gastrointestinal disease and discomfort were
so widespread in infants and toddlers that I began to
feel badly about prescribing what I had been taught
–Donnatal and Sedadrops (atropine, hyoscamine,
alcohol, belladonna, phenobarbital–even opium
derivatives) – and instead began to diagnose what I
called the *"Tube Syndrome."*

New mothers were often so concerned (along with, or because of, stressed fathers) that they lacked parenting skills that they got caught in a maze of fears about feeding their babies, which they did excessively with amazing varieties of food. They worried full time about what food went into the baby – its consistency, amount, flavor, type, temperature, and timing – and what came out of the baby in terms of amount, time, smell, frequency and consistency.

These parents were seeing their babies as tubes that began at the mouth and ended at the anus. To put an end to the *"Tube Syndrome"* took patience. I had to offer constant reasurance and I stopped the medicines for the colic, gas, vomiting and diarrhea, while coaxing the parents to just forget about what was going into and coming out of the baby for a while. "Let Nature take its course," I would tell them as I crossed my fingers and made mental notes to call back every day to check on the baby's status.

When parents began seeing their baby where a *"tube"* had been, they began dispensing the love and nurture that was all the baby wanted in the first place. I found that in times of stress, babies get colic because they swallow air; *and* they swallow air so they can get colic and attention! No matter what our age we require nurture as well as nourishment.

A NEW KIND OF PRACTICE

I was becoming acutely aware of these deficiencies in my medical training, even though the
institutions where I had trained were among the best
in the country and my teachers among the best
(Julius Richmond, M.D., at Upstate Medical
Center of New York and Paul Wehrle, M.D., at the
University of Southern California). It was Wehrle
who had helped lead the successful effort that
virtually wiped out smallpox on the planet, and who
opened up new vistas for me each time he wound up
a lecture on infectious disease by writing a capital
"R" on the blackboard for "resistance to disease,"
he said, a factor about which we knew virtually
nothing; a medical riddle we must someday
unravel.

My training was excellent in diagnostic and
treatment skills. We were taught the profound need
to *"listen with the third ear*," as they called it, to
really listen to what the patient was saying. My
mentors were brilliant and compassionate. They
instilled in all of us a sense of concern for all that we
still did not know or fully understand. Most of all
they instilled a passionate ethic in patient care:
"First, do no harm." What a shock it was to me to
analyze a pratice after twenty years and find myself
spending eighty percent of my time with the
Worried Well and the *Walking Wounded,* who
were seeing me as a *pill fairy(!)* on whom they
depended to stay healthy.

I started a health-promotion and disease-prevention program in my medical clinic – a thriving university-oriented, fee-for-service private group practice in California. With the clinic's health facilitator, my former wife, Serina Taub, R.N., I started teaching more than two thousand children and their families to eat better, exercise regularly, communicate and express feelings more effectively, curtail television watching, set goals and keep journals, and meditate daily.

We talked at great length with the families who, according to our records, were experiencing more than their share of sickness.

We told parents and those children old enough to understand (age four and up) that increased personal responsibility for their health would enhance their self-value and stimulate the release of healing chemicals (endorphins) in their bodies that could help them be well. *We explained that laughter, hope, faith and love were powerful medicines, and that their own minds were the most important force in determining illness or health.*

Children as young as four years old began effectively to set goals and meditate. Children and their families began to keep journals and modify each other's unhealthy behaviors, including smoking, alcohol and drug use. Constructive means of expressing anger and other emotions were played out in households where there had been only violence in words or action.

For thousands of our patients there were

Boy's Prediction of Dying So Ailing Girlfriend Could Have Heart for Transplant Comes True

PATTERSON, Calif. (AP) — A 15-year-old boy who learned his girlfriend needed a heart transplant told his mother three weeks ago that he was going to die and that the young woman should have his heart.

Felipe Garza Jr., who had seemed to be in perfect health, died Saturday after a blood vessel burst in his head.

His family followed his wishes, and Felipe's heart was transplanted Sunday to Donna Ashlock as his last act of love.

His brother, John Sanchez, 20, said Felipe told their mother, Maria, three weeks ago: "I'm going to die, and I'm going to give my heart to my girlfriend."

Donna, 14, who also lived in this farming community 75 miles southeast of San Francisco, had just learned that she had an enlarged heart and needed a transplant.

"I guess they were pretty close," Sanchez said.

He said Felipe complained of pain on the left side of his head when he woke up Saturday morning.

"He was losing breath, and he couldn't walk," Sanchez said.

Garza was taken to the local hospital, then flown to a larger hospital in Modesto, 20 miles away.

But the blood supply to Felipe's brain had been cut off so long by the burst blood vessel that he was brain dead, and remained technically alive only because he had been placed on a respirator, Sanchez added.

The family decided to let physicians remove Felipe's heart for Donna and his kidneys and eyes for others in need of those organs.

"We didn't want to see him suffer no more, and what else could we do?" Sanchez asked.

"It was our decision from what the doctor explained to us. We decided to go ahead and give Donna her heart."

With life-support systems keeping his organs alive, Felipe was flown before dawn Sunday to San Francisco's Presbyterian Hospital, where Donna already was undergoing tests.

A team of surgeons removed Felipe's organs, and Donna got her transplant in a five-hour operation Sunday afternoon.

Dr. J. Donald Hill, who led the transplant team, said the surgery went smoothly.

Donna's condition on Monday improved to good from critical, and doctors removed a breathing tube. Her parents declined to talk with reporters, said hospital spokeswoman Nancy Millhouse.

A dramatic example of the way the mind controls the body.

dramatic changes in health, behavior and attitude, as children and adults learned that praise was an effective form of love. School principals found so-called "hyperactive" children modifying their teachers' expectations. Families were eating well, exercising, meditating and communicating . . . and we were amazed during the three years of the program that the incidence of disease, illness and office visits plummeted dramatically – as much as eighty percent or more. The children were just not getting sick as often, not coming in as frequently, and not requiring all the medicine, surgical procedures, x-rays and lab tests they previously had needed.

Laughter, hope, faith and *love* emerged during the health-promotion program at our clinic as the most potent healing forces.[2]

The "Worried Well" and "Walking Wounded" became truly well because a pediatrician and a health facilitator, one an M.D. and the other a R.N., shifted the patients' beliefs and expectations from illness to *Wellness*. Patients took on new beliefs in the power of their inner healing strength, and new

---

[2]ANATOMY OF AN ILLNESS AS PERCEIVED BY THE PATIENT by Norman Cousins (W.W. Norton, 1979) is a wonderful book about the author's successful campaign against a serious illness. He overcame terrible pain and at least one expert's announcement that his odds for full recovery were only one in five hundred. His weapons in the battle for *Wellness* were faith, hope, love and laughter. ANATOMY OF AN ILLNESS was the first major popular book to demonstrate the importance of the patient's participation in the healing process. I strongly recommend it.

belief in their expectation that they could accomplish almost anything they set their minds to.

About two thousand patients succumbed willingly to the age-old enchantment of the caring and concerned doctor's presence. Shaman, medicine man, healer; the name is not important. What is important is that in a society where the M.D. is regarded as a "*Minor Deity*," that power to impress people can be used as a first step in teaching them to be well. The M.D.'s role then becomes more than an exercise in technology and surgical proficiency; it becomes an inducement to healing and *Wellness*. When Integrative Medicine weds the tools and techniques of modern Western Medicine to all the other healing methods available – including the strength of the patient's own spiritual values – large and small "miracles" do happen every day.

Case History: "A Success Story For You"

Dear Doctor:

Here's a success story for you. After seeing you last month during eight year old David's bout with chicken pox and then for a physical and discussing with you the changes in your practice, I have had time to consider how your ideas might affect changes in our lives.

A review of David's history will serve to refresh your memory regarding his allergies. Although David annually seems to have difficulty with allergies during the fall, his asthma period this year was approaching three months as opposed to two weeks in the past. (I hadn't even been aware of this until you stirred up my thinking!) For the past weeks, David required medication before bed, and without fail would awaken during the night needing more.

One night when I felt especially tired and was tucking David in bed, I said, "David, mom and dad are really tired of getting up every night, so tonight if you wake up just use your mind – the meditation that Doctor Taub taught you – to control your breathing and coughing." He did wake up that night – in fact, three times! But he never called us, and he would be asleep in several minutes. *Mother* had a much rougher time that night than David did, but I didn't go into his room.

And now that you're sitting there saying, "I told you so," you may have guessed that David has had no medicine for the last week, and we all anticipate more and more days and nights medicine-free.

Future changes? Who knows, although I anticipate no more allergy shots. Should that not work out, then we'll alter the path down which we're walking. Share with us in the joy of our mutual success.

(David's mother)

This new kind of medical practice, Integrative Medicine, may be described as a biological, social, psychological, spiritual approach to getting well and staying healthy. In this age of stress, Integrative Medicine demystifies the origins of disease. It draws on the healing systems of other cultures where appropriate. While we recognize the need for distinguished and rigorous medical training, hospitals and technology, the basis of the body of knowledge that is Integrative Medicine is one of *self-help, self-care, self-understanding, self-value* and *self-healing*.

The theory and practices of Integrative Medicine have been presented to the National Academy of Sciences, The American Academy of Pediatrics, The National Education Association, and the American Association of University Women. The medical school deans who were present at the National Academy of Sciences informed me that they had been trying to get medical students to take heed of such precepts of healing for about fifty years, without notable success! Integrative Medicine provided the basis for the Alto-Snowbird Medical Institute in Utah, and *Voyage to Wellness* programs onboard passenger ships such as the Queen Elizabeth II, Sagafjord, Vistafjord, Caribe and Stardancer.

From the theoretical basis of Integrative Medicine comes the process of achieving longer life with higher quality. It is both powerful and practical, and it can affect changes in your life that you never dreamed possible. I have come to think of this process as a *bridge* to *Wellness*, and in the next few chapters I will teach you how to step onto this bridge and continue across until you are on the well side.

Remember that *you* are the most important part of the process. The *bridge* reawakens an always present and indomitable healing force within you.

The precepts of Integrative Medicine are simple and as old as the beginning of recorded history; it is a *psycho-social and bio-spiritual approach to understanding health and dealing with dis-ease.*

The results of crossing the bridge are immediate and long lasting. The most difficult and complex patients I have ever encountered in twenty-five years of practice respond as well as the individuals with less serious difficulty.

Because you must take responsibility for your success on this journey, you can predict your success by examining the degree to which you are willing to take responsibility. The following test is both a predictor of success and a *Wellness* measuring device. Remember there is no right or wrong answer to any of the questions. There is no good or bad—no judgments at all are made. This test simply tells you whether or not and to what degree you are *willing* to be well at this time.

WELLNESS MEASUREMENTS

The response-ability scale and the quotient you derive from it will tell you immediately where you are on your journey to *Wellness*. It all depends on whether your response-ability quotient is anabolic (*life enhancing*) or catabolic (*life destructive*).

To change your lifestyle from catabolic to anabolic requires only the most basic effort of will power and commitment on your part. No matter what your response-ability quotient, you can be on the path to optimal *Wellness* during the next five weeks by following the Prescription For Life—it is your Bridge to *Wellness*.

If your quotient is currently catabolic, you are simply not willing to be well at the present time. *Right now, only great luck and terrific genes can help you.* A catabolic quotient is life destructive, and generally predicts failure to achieve or maintain *Wellness*. The rest of this book can help you understand and change the negative programming that has put you in this position. Maybe tomorrow you will change. Maybe it will take longer. Perhaps you will not want to change. That choice is yours. For everyone, however, the most modest effort to keep in step across the bridge will increase your self-esteem. This in turn will actually improve the flow of healing chemicals in your body which, in turn, improves your chance of success.

Positive and negative answers do not entail right or wrong, good or bad. They are simple no's and yes's. You have the right to your choice, whatever it is.

It will take you five weeks to cross the bridge to *Wellness*, whatever your response-ability quotient is. It generally takes that long to really notice how much better you are feeling. At that point your own psychophysiological (mind and body) *Wellness* circuit will be established and you will know it's your own choice that put you there. Success brings more success, and your healthy patterns grow.

YOUR RESPONSE-ABILITY SCALE

The response-ability scale measures your ability to respond to moment-to-moment choices in your life that are significant in terms of your health. Mark the categories on the response-ability scale that describe you best. Use common sense if you are unsure of any answers. Leave unmarked any statements that do not apply to you.

Your choices are either anabolic or catabolic. Anabolism and catabolism are regarded as positive or negative, but not good or bad. One builds up; the other breaks down. Just as spring builds up and fall breaks down, so your choices are natural and neutral; neither good nor bad. *There should never be guilt or blame attached to illness.* When we turn our back on positive choices it is a reflection of the overwhelming stress that caused our difficulty in the first place. Judgment is not implied by anabolic/catabolic.

Whatever your ability to respond to the choices in your life, remember it is always your choice to continue at your present level or to move toward a more or less healthy lifestyle. *The choice is always yours.*

The Taub
Response-Ability Scale

ANABOLIC CHOICES

( ) I DON'T SMOKE

( ) I DON'T ABUSE ALCOHOL OR DRUGS

( ) I GENERALLY EXERCISE REGULARLY AND FEEL FAIRLY PHYSICALLY FIT

( ) I AM ABOUT THE RIGHT WEIGHT AND I EAT FAIRLY SENSIBLY

( ) I AM CONNECTED TO OTHERS IN MEANINGFUL FRIENDSHIPS OR LOVING RELATIONSHIPS

( ) I AM ESSENTIALLY A POSITIVE PERSON, ENJOY LAUGHING AND HAVE FAITH THAT THINGS WILL BE OK

( ) I USE SEAT BELTS AND AM A SAFE DRIVER

( ) I GENERALLY FEEL WELL

CATABOLIC CHOICES

( )   I SMOKE

( )   I ABUSE ALCOHOL OR DRUGS

( )   I RARELY, IF EVER, EXERCISE; I AM NOT VERY FIT

( )   I AM DEFINITELY UNDER OR OVER-WEIGHT AND I AM NOT VERY SENSIBLE ABOUT HOW I EAT

( )   I HAVE NO REAL MEANINGFUL FRIEND-SHIPS OR LOVING RELATIONSHIPS

( )   I AM GENERALLY NEGATIVE; I RARELY LAUGH AND I DON'T SEE A LOT OF REASONS FOR OPTIMISM

( )   I DON'T USE SEAT BELTS OR DRIVE VERY SAFELY

( )   GENERALLY, I JUST DON'T FEEL PARTICULARLY WELL

YOUR RESPONSE-ABILITY QUOTIENT

Determine your response-ability quotient by adding up the number of anabolic answers you checked and subtracting from that total the number of catabolic answers you checked.

Example: If you had six anabolic and two catabolic answers, subtract two from six for a responsibility quotient of *four*.

WHAT IT MEANS

If your response-ability quotient is **6-8** you have excellent health potential.

If your response-ability quotient was **4-6** you have average health potential.

A responses-ability quotient of **2-4** means you have poor health potential.

A response-ability quotient of **0-2** shows that your survival is a matter of luck and good genes.

A response-ability quotient (RQ) of **six** (one catabolic answer) indicates, for all practical purposes, you are in a state of optimal *Wellness*. You have taken charge of your health destiny. You are a person of strength and conviction and recognize the power of your choices. You are personally responsible for yourself, have a good sense of self-value and high regard for life. Your PRESCRIPTION FOR LIFE will involve changing your sole negative response to a positive one. It may seem difficult to be "perfect," but those of you with this high a responsibility quotient will find it to be easy.

An RQ of **four** (two catabolic answers) shows you are about as well as most people who are feeling good about themselves. You have taken responsibility for your health and well being and have developed a sufficiently high regard for life to want to look and feel as good as you can. It is important to get yourself on the bridge to *Wellness* and develop a higher RQ. Your two negative answers could be a keg of dynamite. Your goal will be to change at least one catabolic answer to an anabolic one.

An RQ of **two** (three catabolic answers) indicates a lifestyle and behavior pattern generally consistent with low self-esteem and a sense of just giving up on life as too tough to cope with. Continuing at this level puts you in the winter of your existence, the twilight instead of the dawn. The key for you is your willingness to increase your RQ with more anabolic choices for life. You can experience dramatic and life-saving changes by getting on the bridge to *Wellness* immediately. By taking the steps across the bridge to *Wellness*, you will find it easy to change at least one of your negative responses to a positive one.

An RQ of **0** (four catabolic answers) indicates that you are *willing* yourself to deterioration and death. Overt change in your social behavior and lifestyle is *crucial* if you are to survive. Your attitudes and strength can be enhanced by taking the first step on the bridge. Your life can be turned around if you are willing to construct a health agreement for the bridge. If you will move up to an RQ of at least four, by turning around two of your negative patterns, you will change your health destiny. The choice is yours to make either way. The steps across the bridge will help you change at least two of your answers on the response-ability scale.

Here is a quicker and more concise way to also measure your *Wellness*. You can take this test in less than a minute to determine your present health and measure your health potential. None of the questions on this test have to do with being sick. This is a *Wellness* test.

Dr. Taub's "Life Choices" Test

☐   I don't smoke.

☐   I don't abuse alcohol or drugs

☐   I excercise regularly, and feel fairly fit.

☐   I am about the right weight and I'm sensible about what I eat.

☐   I am connected with others through meaningful friendships or loving relationships.

☐   I am essentially a positive person, enjoy laughing, and have faith things will be okay.

☐   I use seat belts, and I am a safe driver

☐   I am generally healthy and feel well.

Here is the way the test is graded. Give yourself one point for every true statement about yourself.

YOUR SCORE ☐

To score
"Life Choices" test

7-8:   You have excellent health potential.

5-6:   You have average health potential

3-4:   You have poor health potential.

0-2:   Your survival is a matter of luck and good genes.

Now that you have seen where you are and how far the bridge to *Wellness* will take you, I will explain how to positively program your psychological and physiological factors to work for you when you are on the bridge.

Chapter Four

The "S Factor"

SMOULDERING STRESS SYNDROME

In addition to the major stresses of our personal lives (deaths, births, marriages, mortgages, jobs, divorces) to which we might logically react, we are bombarded today with thousands of environmental stresses.

Stress has become ever-present in our lives through the media in the form of sad and bad news, through advertising, violence in songs, movies and TV, through competitiveness in fashion, politics, sports, and with neighbors, and through programming in school, church, doctors' offices, at work and even at home where threats and warnings are used for motivation.

A constant mental as well as physical bombardment of aggravation, hassle and annoyance has caused what I call "The Smouldering Stress Syndrome," or more simply, the "S Factor." It is the modern descendant of what Hans Selye called the "general adaptation syndrome" of stress.

Selye was the first to explain the "fight or flight" response to stress. This is the body's natural way to get ready to either fight whatever is causing the stress or to "run like hell" to get away from it. Our breathing quickens, our adrenalin flows faster, and other biochemical changes take place to prepare us to face whatever threatens.

Selye went on to explore what happens when the body misconstrues the minor stresses of daily life, magnifying them physically as if they were life-threatening. The result is a burden on the adrenal system and the rest of the body that it was never intended to bear.

Today's ever-present stress continues, and our reactions to the stress persists long after the immediate stimulus is over. We never give our bodies a chance to get back to their unstressed, neutral positions. Once we are upset, we do not get back to the base line or "zero" before something else happens to disturb our bodies or psyches.

As this never-ending stress remains and we continue to react to stress that is not clearly visible long after the stress cause is gone, the result is an internal dilemma that adds to the stress. We think, *"Nothing wrong is happening, but I feel terrible."* This leads to *more* confusion and anxiety which just leads to more stress—the slow, simmering, *smouldering* pressure that I call the "S Factor."

What was once a real reaction to a real threatening situation (the fight or flight response to stress) itself has now become a threat to our lives through degenerative diseases. This cycle of stress that causes stress that causes stress is a sly plague. Until the plague becomes life-threatening, we tend to ignore its silent onset.

The "S Factor" has become the dominant theme in our society. It is most evident in the rapid destruction of family values, moral codes, education and the environment.

Family values have eroded with as many divorces as marriages; there are more children in day-care centers or left alone during the day than with their parents; we have more fast food treats than family meals; more role models for life are being provided by television soap operas and violent movies than by families and schools.

Morals have deteriorated with pornography and explicit sexual material that is rampant and overwhelming—in books, television, movies, songs, magazines, billboards and newspapers—and we are conditioned to believe "authorities" who explain that this does not lead to an increase in murder, rape, kidnapping and child molestation. Even in Family or PG rated movies, the "coming attractions" now convey images of simulated sex acts.

So silent is the onset of the "S Factor" and the changes in our societies folkways, that the list of the top seven problems confronting our schools according to the March 17, 1988 Dear Abby column, has changed in the following ways:

TOP PROBLEMS

1940	1988
1-Talking	1-Drug Abuse
2-Chewing Gum	2-Alcohol Abuse
3-Making Noises	3-Pregnancy
4-Running in the Halls	4-Suicide
5-Getting Out of Line	5-Rape
6- Improper Clothing	6-Robbery
7-Not Putting Paper in the Wastebaskets	7-Assault

Educational values and goals have changed dramatically. There has been a de-emphasis in the development of character, honesty and ethical behaviour. The teaching of classical music, art, dance, literature and poetry has been downgraded. We are not creating a working knowledge of history and geography in our schools. The tendency today is towards graduating computer-functional students who are illiterate in life. A 1988 survey of 180 school children, ages 7-12, in the Washington D.C. surburban Maryland area, showed that they could name an average of only 4.8 United States Presidents—but that they could name an average of 5.2 brands of beer!

A good deal of high technology and science is destroying our environment and threatening the very existence of our planet; it is poisoning our sun's rays, acidifying our rain, destroying our forests, heating our weather, increasing our droughts, changing the tides, ruining our oceans and polluting our air. Our entire planet can be blown up several times over in only a few seconds with all of the weapons now being stored by big and little countries. Talk about stress!

The "S Factor," this *smouldering stress syndrome,* reaches remarkable levels. It simmers and smoulders in us until it becomes a heap of anxiety, resentment, fear and worry. It grows into a critical mass of negative energy that is able to cause dis-ease. The "S Factor" builds up enough negative energy to interfere with the powerful healing forces of the body. When this occurs, blueprints or genetic templates of disease (described in the next section of this book), emerge prematurely and our thoughts get out-of-control. The "S Factor" causes the mind to believe sick and tired thoughts that eventually become so powerful that they attack and destroy the very person *thinking* them in the first place. *This is how mind cancer takes root.*

Constant stress, is so often the key that opens our bodies to the possibility of illness, it becomes urgent that we learn to recognize it, control it, and disarm it. We can disarm it because our personal stress is still *a result* of our reaction and response to what is happening around us. Stress is merely our *perception* of the people and circumstances in our lives. Our stress is based on our *appraisal* of our ability to cope. *Stress begins between our ears!*

MIND CANCER

The "S Factor" spawns an area in the mind that gets out of control—a cancer. Physical cancer results when normal cells change or mutate to enable them to proliferate and grow wildly out of all control. These runaway mutant cells infiltrate or cause pressure to overpower and kill neighboring cells and organs. These cells also travel throughout the body, detroying and attacking. Cancers arising from different cells act differently. Some destroy locally and others kill fast. Curiously, some people have identical cancers and yet react entirely differently; one patient may be affected very minimally while another is devastated; one patient may respond extremely well to treatment while another may not respond at all.

Scientists have traditionally viewed cancer as a physical disease causing deterioration of the body. Cancer, however, from the viewpoint of Integrative Medicine is a deterioration due to an imbalance of the entire organism—body, mind and spirit. *An entire person has cancer, not just his or her liver, pancreas or spleen.*

Recall the scientist's definition of cancer: the proliferation of cells that grow wild and destroy and attack. Now substitute "thoughts" for "cells." Mind cancer becomes the *proliferation of thoughts* that grow wild and destroy and attack. Can you see that when our thoughts and attitudes become twisted because of worry, fear and anger, the very same thing as body cancer occurs in our mind as

our optimism, tranquility and joy are destroyed?
When there is physical cancer, there is *always* mind
cancer—*and one can lead to the other*. Just as
water is steam and ice at the same time, so too is
body, mind and spirit.

Mind cancer has become the most prevalent
form of illness in this age of the "S Factor" and its
ascendancy to power. Here is what mind cancer can
cause—beginning with the "A's": Alzheimers,
anger, alcoholism, anxiety, arthritis, addiction,
atherosclerosis, anorexia and AIDS.

THE TEMPLATES OF DISEASE

Within your cellular structure, the DNA (the
substance of genes) contains templates, or blueprints,
of all the characteristics and body types, strengths
and powers, diseases and genetic factors of your
mother, father, grandparents and ancestors from the
very beginning.

Your resistance to the physical or mental
expression of the harmful templates decreases at
various periods and ages of your life. Conversely,
the potential of your beneficial templates *increases*
when you assume certain lifestyles, attitudes,
convictions and values.

Stress is the key that unlocks the "vaults" in
which your harmful templates are normally safely
stored under the healing and balancing forces of
your body. Some of these vaults are called
ribosomes.

Since stress releases life-destroying templates

prematurely, you can, by reducing stress, reposition the templates of disease safely back in the vaults to remain dormant for long periods of time, perhaps always.

Rheumatoid Arthritis is a good example of the way templates work. What I describe now, however, is the same, in principle, for diabetes, hypertension, coronary artery disease, multiple sclerosis, asthma, allergy, ileitis, colitis, schizophrenia, migraine, backache, peptic ulcer, Alzheimers disease, AIDS, cancer or virtually any other disease. Actually, whatever name we choose to call an illness, the bottom line is that it is a state of dis-ease, an imbalance of body, mind and spirit.

Rheumatoid Arthritis would most likely affect you if you were a woman in your twenties or thirties. And if it did, it would occur in you in the same manner and pattern that it would have occurred elsewhere in your family, even in a great-great-great-great-great aunt, many generations past.

The disease would begin as a redness, warmth and swelling with pain and limitation of movement in the middle joints of your fingers. Your disease would then spread to your wrist joints which would become hot and painful to touch and cause your hands to turn inward as you tried to rest them in your lap, until one day you would find your hands turned that way permanently because of destruction of the wrist joint space. The destruction would be occurring as a result of your own immune system creating antibodies to your own body.

Yes, you make antibodies with which to *attack*

yourself; antibodies that inflame, ravage and demolish not only your joints, but your blood, your marrow, your liver and spleen, your kidney and eyes, and eventually every organ in your system. In the case of Rheumatoid Arthritis, after the hands began turning inward, the joints around the mouth and jaw, the temporal mandibular joints, would begin to cause the face to assume a long, drawn out, depressive looking expression that becomes frozen as the bodily destruction continues.

Simultaneously, the inner organs – liver, kidney, spleen, blood vessels, the blood itself, the retina of the eyes, begin undergoing characteristic and predictable changes. Now here is what is amazing about all of this: whether observed with the naked eye or confirmed by microscope, x-rays, blood or urine tests, *all these changes would be the same changes that had occurred in the great-great-great-great-great aunt or any similarly afflicted relatives. You would have inherited the same genetic material, the same DNA that incorporated the blueprint or template of the disease.*

Rheumatoid Arthritis is described in thousands of medical texts as a generalized autoimmune disease that attacks the certain finger joints and the wrist, face, and organs in the most characteristic and peculiar ways; *the description is accurate because the body must follow the programs of its genetic templates.*

Depending on your ancestry, you might have templates for chronic respiratory disease (emphysema, bronchitis, lung cancer in adults, and

colds, ear infections, tonsillitis, asthma in children)
– or diabetes, gout, ileitis, colitis, stomach cancer,
hemorroids, psoriasis, eczema, acne, cystitis,
migraine, pyelonephritis, etc. Under constant
stress, these templates become the hallmarks of the
Walking Wounded and the *Worried Well.*

Despite the fact that your DNA contains all the
diseases, weaknesses, and detrimental factors of
your inheritance, you yourself are generally without
illness most of your days. This is incredible when
you consider that the templates for all of the
diseases of your ancestors are in the DNA of all
your trillions of cells and that those cells then divide
into other cells carrying the same templates over
and over and over again. *Why aren't you just
constantly, totally just "walking disease?"*

Your cells have another substance within them
called "Messenger RNA" that literally transports
the genetic messages that are encoded in the DNA.
The "Messenger RNA" carries the genetic messages
to the little power-houses of your cells called
ribosomes. The ribosomes then manufacture proteins
that are based on the genetic messages.

According to the genetic messages (or templates)
your ribosomes produce the protein that makes up
the substance of all your new cells. The message
may transmit a template that says *"make red
pigment and curl-producing elasticity for the
hair,"* or *"disrupt hair follicle growth when this
body reaches age forty-five,"* or *"initiate the
pattern of Rheumatoid Arthritis."* Curly redheads,
bald men or Rheumatoid Arthritis—it all starts with

templates.

Taking the example a step further now, you should be able to imagine that each of your cells, when it divides into two more, is also transmitting all of its encoded template messages. Actually then, each new cell in you has the template for virtually all the deteriorating factors, from Rheumatoid Arthritis to baldness, that your ancestors ever had.

The reason *you* are not totally and continuously diseased is that the healing force that scientists call *homeostasis* is within you. It keeps your *life-destructive* templates safely dormant. Homeostasis *neutralizes* disease templates so you do not become ill. Additionally, homeostasis encourages the activity of the *life-enhancing* templates that keep you healthy and well.

The means by which homeostasis blocks the activity of *life-destructive* templates is not generally known or understood. It certainly goes beyond our traditional understanding of dominant and recessive genes. The template theory is based on our present knowledge of another substance in the cells called "Suppressor RNA" and our medical understanding of the effects of stress on the body.

"Suppressor RNA" is able to *block* the transport of encoded template messages by either preventing the "Messenger RNA" from reaching the protein factories in your cells, or by preventing the encoded template messages on your DNA from being carried by the "Messenger RNA" in the first place.

The key to the template theory may be "Suppressor RNA." If it is efficient and if there is enough of it, it should be able to either block "Messenger RNA" on its journey or deter the templates from being carried by "Messenger RNA." Thus your ancestral deterioration factors just remain dormant, and let you live in an anabolic or life-enhancing state. "Suppressor RNA" may actually be the major factor contributing to the still somewhat mysterious process of homeostasis. Constant stress can disrupt the function of "Suppressor RNA" and allow the templates of disease to come out of the vaults in which they are usually safely kept. *Neutralizing stress can allow disease templates to be safely "locked-up" once more.*

The same Dr. Hans Selye who first put forth the theory of the fight or flight response to stress also demonstrated that every single cell, organ, and system in the human body will react and respond to constant threats in the environment, including ongoing concerns to the mind and continuous attacks (nutritional, environmental and others) on the body. Selye showed that physical exhaustion, immunological breakdown, and eventual adrenal collapse can result from prolonged stress.

The template theory of disease postulates that stress from detrimental lifestyle, unhealthy thoughts and beliefs (especially involving fear, insecurity, hopelessness, depression, anger, grief or resentment) actually acts to weaken or block the "Suppressor RNA," and allows destructive, catabolic templates to emerge prematurely, and in many instances unnecessarily.

The template theory recognizes the immense physical, emotional and environmental stress we live under and the role of the *smouldering stress syndrome* — The "S Factor"—that constantly attacks our bodies, minds and spirits.

The reason so many people are in the legions of the *Walking Wounded* and *Worried Well*, may be due to destructive templates emerging *prematurely* because of the effects of stress on "Suppressor RNA." The results of physical, emotional, mental and environmental stress are evident in the whole range of our misery from colds to cancer, and arthritis to AIDS.

Key points to remember, as you marshall your self to cross "the bridge from sick and tired" to *Wellness* are these:

1. As long as tissue death has not occurred, any illness is potentially reversible because of your remarkable healing forces and the power of your mind and body to make you well.

2. Stress is causing destructive templates to emerge prematurely—in many cases unnecessarily. Stress is the key that unlocks the "vaults" containing harmful templates of disease.

The techniques you will learn on your way to *Wellness* will enable you to reduce stress and safely return disease templates to the "vault" where they belong. Remember, stress essentially begins between your ears!

CANCER IS A GENETIC DISEASE

"Genetics May Play Role in Colon Cancer,
Researchers Find"   September 1, 1988
                                    Los Angeles Times

I am continuously surprised to see headlines like the above, because almost *all* disease patterns are locked into genetic codes.

Codes or templates determine how the body responds and why one body generally responds similarly to another body with the same disease—whether it be diabetes, migraine or colon cancer.

The templates or blueprints are ways that the body is programmed in predictable patterns to deteriorate. This is nature's own *"self-destruct mechanism."* Living forms eventually expire so new life can take their place.

Some cancers spread only locally doing damage by causing pressure on surrounding tissues—pancreatic cancer destroys in this way. This is because pancreatic cancer cells are genetically programmed to behave in a certain fashion—that is to spread locally. Perhaps the rest of the body is also programmed to *resist* generalized spreading of pancreas cancer cells.

Cancers of the lung, prostate, uterus, intestines or breast behave differently from pancreas cancer *and* from each other. They *do* spread elsewhere; they spread to different organs and different places in the body—some spread to the bones or the brain, others to the blood or the marrow. It is all predictable! *Cancers differ according to their templates or genetic codes, the behaviour of the cancer cells as well as the response of the body is predictible.* Thus, cancer is a genetic disease, one of the templates of dis-ease through which the body breaks down along predetermined patterns when it becomes stressed or is just ready to die.

Since templates of disease are dormant or suppressed by the forces in our body called homeostasis, we could lead relatively dis-ease free lives until we pass on as part of Nature's plan. Unfortunately however, the vast percentage of our disease now occurs prematurely and short circuits our potential for longer life. You will see more and more headlines like the one for colon cancer announcing that genes are behind it. *Of course they are!*

LIFE PROMOTERS

In countering stress and following the Prescription For Life, there are certain *life-promoting* forces at your disposal.

Life Promoter Number 1: AT-ONE-MENT

Integrative Medicine incorporates an acceptance that life energy never dies; it merely takes other forms. This is in accordance with the principle in physics that states that matter cannot be created or destroyed.

The human body is an incredible example of motion and energy in balance. With the natural aging process, certain factors will emerge as the templates of disease are sifted by Nature assessing her choices to replenish herself.

Like a field of flowers, we must eventually make room for other lives to grow. But as the energy of the flowers goes right back into the soil to replenish it and help produce next season's splendor, so too does our life energy go on in one form or another after death—a cloud, a drop of dew, a rainbow, some sunshine, perhaps an angel.

A corollary of this acceptance of life and death is that faith, *merely a willingness to believe*, just a simple respect and reverence for life itself, is the greatest healing factor known to man. Integrative Medicine accepts that spectacular cures often occur in the human body left to its own devices when all else fails. Not even the Mayo Clinic can match the recuperative power of the most primitive elementary cell in the human body. The lowliest cell, say a cell producing the cuticle for your left fifth fingernail, has more intelligence and is more complicated than the computer we devised to send satellites and people into space and bring them back.

Integrative Medicine encourages patients to have faith and to take time to turn silently inward to one's own concept of life-energy, Nature, a Higher Power or God. Not with a sense of guilt or sin or atonement! These are often our own mistaken concepts. But with peacefulness, lovingness, goodness, caring, gratitude and reverence. When we learn to turn inward, to quiet the mind and just let nature do the rest, we strengthen the anabolic, life-enhancing systems that keep us well. Quieting the mind when we turn inward helps us erase the effects of all the negative forces in our lives: the physical, mental, emotional and spiritual stresses and feelings that take their toll. You may have been taught to *think,* by people who have erroneously interpreted their religious faith into "churches of universal guilt," that your life should be spent in atonement. This is just not so. The basis of *all* the major faiths involve a "oneness" with God, Nature, Love and all living things. When we turn inward and just let Nature be, we experience a *connectedness* to all of life. As our respect for that connection grows, our health improves. This spiritual connection need not be theologically based. It is simply an acceptance of love and forgiveness and a rejection of guilt and punishment. It is not atonement. It is *at-one-ment.* An important part of the Prescription For Life is this turning silently inward. You are capable of learning how to develop this reverence for life, which is, in itself, the major life-promoting, healing catalyst for *Wellness.*

Life Promoter Number 2: Confluent Events

In learning to let go of the burden of stress, it is helpful to be acquainted with the idea of the meaningful composition of events. This is the idea that events are always flowing together for the positive or the negative or, as we would usually term it, the good or the bad, the ill or the well.

When you look at events and circumstances, you see only a small part of the picture. Some people find inner peace from their belief that a Higher Power or Supreme Being sees the entire picture and directs a confluence of multiple events so that in the larger picture, it all turns out for the good.

Today, when stress is behind virtually every disease, the consequence of this belief is overwhelmingly important. Since the greatest cause of stress is the fear and anxiety underlying our thoughts, a belief that it is all for a greater good can alleviate the stress that our thoughts induce.

Integrative Medicine accepts the idea of confluent events, which is similiar to the Eastern teaching of the law of *karma*, or the Western notion of *"as you sow, so you shall reap."* Whatever good thoughts you have will come back to you in good ways. Whatever *Wellness* producing thoughts you have will come back to you as *Wellness*. And, of course, the same would be true if you thought negatively and thought illness producing thoughts.

Many people will scoff at this idea, but I have

seen it in practice over and over again. The people who will laugh at this concept, those who "*know better*" because they are "*experts*," tend to be the people who are running our stress filled society: scientists, corporate officers, advertising executives, munitions manufacturers, military officers, politicians—all the people who are programming us for stress, by creating and controlling our environment, influencing our world and contributing to the current dismal state of our planet.

Just because you can't prove something scientifically doesn't mean that it is not so! I would have had difficulty in medical school if I professed this belief then, but there is a lot that cannot be validated scientifically. Unfortunately, Western science leaves little room for the human experience. There is so much that we do not understand, but this does not mean that more than what we know does not exist.

You might find it interesting to read about Socrates in this book's physicians information section. He was executed for proclaiming how ignorant we are of our ignorance.

If we are looking only at the underside of a lovely tapestry, we may be seeing only tattered knots. And our lives will reflect that one-sided, wrong-sided view. We will feel disconnected, out of sorts, as if something is wrong. But if we have knowledge of and faith in the existence of the overall beauty of the tapestry, our lives will reflect and encompass beautiful health, beautiful *Wellness* and a feeling that all is right with the world. Feelings and realities will emerge from our beliefs, positive or negative. According to your belief, attitude, conviction and faith, the end results of the confluence of events will be the enhancement of life or the deterioration of life.

Often, we just cannot understand or accept why loved ones, even children die; as a *Wellness* physician, I believe that their souls are merely closer to the heart of God or even dwelling *within* God's heart.

The sadness and hurtful memory of friends and loved ones is only ours. We can remember the loveliness of the person just as we remember last year's flowers and let the memory evoke not sadness, hurt and doubt, but reverence for life and love for Nature or God.

The real meaning of why seemingly bad things happen to good people is only that sometimes we cannot see the overall pattern — only the knots on the underside of the universal tapestry. What causes our mental anguish and stress, whether it is illness, loss of a loved one, a lost opportunity, or anything else is a short-sightedness; an unfamiliarity with the overall pattern of the tapestry. It is no wonder life seems overwhelmingly burdensome to people who perceive it with only themselves and their own perspective as the center of it all! It is the connectedness and faith in the larger picture that alleviates the stress of isolation. You will learn how to recognize and accept this connectedness as a result of the Prescription for Life.

Life Promoter Number 3: Endorphins

Today, research laboratories have identified hundreds of brain-secreted chemicals. Just a few years ago only a few such chemicals were known.

A major part of the body's natural healing system is made up of simple and complex polypeptide chemicals, or clusters of amino acids that the brain secretes. There are hundreds or perhaps thousands of these chemicals. Some of these polypeptides are called endorphins.

Endorphins are part of an extraordinarily powerful, natural defense system. Endorphins and similiar substances help dissolve feelings of discord and dissonance. They enhance our feelings of well-being. Modern science is just beginning to appreciate the benefits of these "feel good" polypeptides.

The so-called "runner's high" is attributed to an increased flow of endorphins. So are the beneficial effects of meditation or the relaxation response. The brain secretes endorphins most efficiently when it is in the alpha or theta state. Our brains are in the alpha or theta state when there is little or no movement of thought: upon waking, just as we fall asleep, when we quiet the mind in meditation or while running; when we are quietly gazing at the stars; whenever our mental "chitchat" is turned off.

Unless you practice quieting the mind, you hardly ever experience times when your brain is not talking at you, planning, worrying, reflecting, remembering or wondering. *The stressful times we live in deprive our brains of silent intervals.* This lack of quietness impedes the abundant flow of endorphins.

To relax completely, to quiet the mind, and to stimulate the production and release of endorphins, one of the oldest techniques is still the best. It is free, it is easy to learn, and every society that has ever existed has used it in one form or another.

To Eastern spiritual masters it is meditation. To Western physicians and psychobiologists, it is the relaxation response. To the spiritually inclined it is the combination of structured prayer and faith.

Whatever you call it, there is nothing mystical about the physiological effects of meditation, relaxation or prayer. (*You don't even have to live in Southern California to do it*!) In a few minutes, you can quiet your mind, stop the flow of thoughts, discontinue the mental "chitchat," and allow the endorphins to do their work.

A feeling of at-one-ment, an understanding of confluent events, exercise, good food and meditation all help to quiet the mind; they help the healing process as they help you take a break from the constant mind chatter that is itself so stressful; they increase the flow of healing, "feel good" endorphins.

Now that you understand some of the techniques and beliefs involved in healing, we will examine the heart of the whole healing process — *life energy.*

Chapter Five

Understanding Life Energy

I n order to understand how our bodies change while following the Prescription For Life, we have to move beyond our image of the body as a collection of cells and organs. The key to understanding this is life energy.

The human body is much more than a collection of trillions of cells and thousands of organs that continuously fall into disrepair. The human body, like all matter, is energy. Understanding this is important to crossing the bridge from sick and tired to *Wellness.*

The real reason Medicine is not working as well as it should is that it is *stuck* at the cellular level. It is stuck fast, because the cellular view leads to the *expectation* that everything in the body, those trillions of cells, will predictably and understandably become disrupted and in need of repair. This expectation is a self-fulfilling prophecy (remember illness-inducing thoughts). And it has been fulfilled to the tune of five hundred billion dollars a year!

Medicine is just where atomic physics would be without the discovery that the old model of the atom as a circle with electrons and protons swarming about a nucleus was just a theory that worked, but only up to a point. At that point atomic physics got stuck. It couldn't progress any further. But even in its incorrect basis, the science made outstanding and world-shaking strides. (More for the bad than the good, it seems now, as we continue to manufacture war machinery that gets more and more powerful. *Each bomb we manufacture today has the equivalent explosive power of the Hiroshima bomb being dropped each and every day for thirteen years).*

There are some striking similarities between misspent atomic energy that destroys instead of builds, and misguided medical care that directs all of its efforts to repair of disease instead of also preventing its onset.

Atomic physicists now understand that the atom and its electrons and protons are not really particles in orbit. Rather, like all matter, they are vibrations, light waves. All matter may be nothing more than light; vibrations, motion in one particular density or another. *In other words, all matter is simply energy.*

Everything we see, breathe, touch, wear, or eat, at its most basic level is energy. Our bodies and minds and brain waves and thoughts are all energy. Just as little drops of water make puddles, streams, rivers and oceans, so do little waves of energy make up our human bodies and our thoughts. (And we have the same choices with our bodies and our thoughts as we do with the world's waterways: we can pollute them, dam them, or let them flow, witness their strength and beauty and derive joy

from them.) We may even just be octillions of tiny
light waves that make up one big wave, one mass of
light energy that we call the body. We are energy.

When we understand that we are energy and not
just cells and organs, we can start to really
understand, perhaps for the first time, how to take
care of ourselves. Just as the mothers who stopped
thinking of their babies as tubes began to see them
as loving beings and knew instinctively how to care
for those babies, so too when we understand life
energy as the true basis of our lives and our health, we
will know very easily what is good for our energy and
what is bad. We will recognize quite simply what is
native to our energy and we will know when a
foreign energy has invaded our own. We will
automatically begin to experience a new awareness
of everything we think, eat, breathe, or are exposed
to in our environment.

When we understand life energy, we will
gravitate toward that which enhances our life
energy. These energy factors are what truly
determine and balance our entire system. The world
we inhabit offers us boundless opportunities for
enhancing our life energy. The Prescription for Life
helps you recognize those things that rob you of
your energy, and those that enhance your energy.
You will learn how to stay well by making choices
that enhance your life energy.

The British scientist A. S. Eddington, writing
fifty years ago in *The Nature of the Physical
World*, described what scientists had been trying to
dig up about the nature of matter during the

preceding one hundred years:

"We have chased solid substance from the continuous liquid to the atom, from the atom to the electron, and there we have lost it."

On what the electron is doing inside the atom, Eddington summarized:

"Something somewhere is doing we don't know what. . ."

Now we know "what"–it is manifesting itself as energy. The next generation of health care will have to consider resonance, frequency, wavelength, harmonics, polarization and energy balance as descriptive terms for bodies that are ill or are well. Physicians will come to understand illness as disharmony, static, dissonance, discord, short-circuiting, cacophony, lack of resonance.

Paradoxically, Eastern Medicine, which Western scientists are only now coming to appreciate, has long understood what we are now testing empirically about life energy. The concept of "ki" (energy) is central to Eastern Medicine, and has been for thousands of years.

I hope I have made it clear that the body is more than a collection of cells and organs that require constant pharmaceutical, psychological and surgical repair. The body is more like an orchestra playing a symphony of resonating tones and vibrations in every cell and throughout its entire system. It is the absence of harmony, (dissonance and discord), that leads to disease and deterioration; not cellular inadequacy or weakness of the organs.

Understanding the body as energy enables us to

choose *Wellness* more easily. We can more easily recognize and neutralize erroneous mental and physical programming, and more easily recognize what outside energy is most compatible with our own. If our body is an orchestra, and beautiful music is our health, then even the little aches and pains, colds and headaches can be tuned out. When every instrument is in perfect pitch, and when we take a few mintues daily to admire the music and care for the instruments, when we stop to really listen, and really hear the music, (for what is a musical instrument, but a vehicle for vibrations?!) we will be enriched physically, emotionally and spiritually. We will be truly and joyfully well.

I want to point out emphatically that the energy and light wave concepts I describe here is at a very early stage of understanding in Western Medicine. Yet is is significantly closer to truth in terms of achieving health and *Wellness* than the earlier, simple theories we have been dealing with. Until now, our theories have generally been leading us safely to disease repair. With an understanding of energy systems we can get well and stay well as whole human beings, not parts that need fixing as they break down or wear out.

Now that we understand that we are made of energy, it is easy to understand how disruptions in our energy can cause dis-ease.

FOREIGN ENERGY

When we understand that illness and disease are an imbalance in our energy, we become aware of some very important self-help measures in preventing and combatting the particular problems that we label infection, allergy, addiction, metabolic difficulties and obesity.

An infection is an example of a foreign energy. There is a germ with its own vibration or frequency or wavelength, intruding upon and interfering with your own natural energy pattern. The interference is what we think of as illness. Your off-balance energy generates the heat we call *fever*; moisture and swelling begin to form in your system and we call them *congestion*; water starts to seep out of you in the form of *perspiration*; your whole system begins to shake and vibrate and rock when your energy is out-of-phase, and you have *chills*.

Look again at the description of infections: Your body is racked with fever or rocked by chills. Doesn't it remind you of a boiler or radiator that clangs, whistles, bangs, steams and either breaks down or blows up? Or of a car that needs its motor tuned, wheels aligned, oil filter replaced, spark plugs changed? How about a washing machine jumping and spinning around while stuck in one cycle and overflowing soap and suds? All of these are energy systems too, and like the human body, they get out of balance.

But nothing is like the human body in its self-healing abilities! We have a built-in system that constantly seeks balance. All we have to do to make it work perfectly is to stop interfering with its innate movement toward balance. It may sound like "New Age" or California language, but we have to learn to just let the energy flow! We have to stop erecting dams that block that energy, and we have to dismantle the dams we have been building for years: negative thought patterns, detrimental lifestyles and injurious habits.

Besides germs, the other common foreign energies that invade and disrupt our own energy are: toxins, microwaves, tobacco, alcohol, drugs, radiation, preservatives, salt, refined sugars, insecticides and even the energy from power lines. Imagine for a moment that when your body is healthy and well, it is like a perfectly functioning television tube with a wonderfully clear picture on the screen. (Televisions! Washing machines! Our bodies are beginning to sound like appliance shops! Who ever heard of an orchestra in an appliance shop?!) The tubes, wires, fuses, and transistors are working in harmony; the focus, contrast and brightness controls and the ones for horizontal and vertical hold are adjusted perfectly; there is no snow or static or fuzziness or glitches in the televisions pictures. The entire energy system is in balance.

Now imagine what happens when you plug in a hair dryer next to the television set. Static, snow, wildly gyrating patterns on the screen. Everything gets fuzzy. Strange noises begin. Everything goes haywire because of energy interference. A foreign energy, an incompatible wavelength or frequency has intruded into and interfered with the energy normally emitted by the television. That disruption in energy is reflected on the screen as glitches, a series of light waves and images that interfere with the images from the TV set.

This analogy is helpful in understanding infection as energy that is out of balance. The analogy is also useful in explaining allergy, addiction, metabolic disease and obesity. The streptococcus germ that looks foreboding as a chain of dots under the microscope, and menacing as a greenish-white growth oozing on a throat culture, is only energy – light waves bound together in a peculiar way determined by the germs' genes and DNA. The light waves bundle together and interact to form the patterns we see microscopically and on the culture, but what it still boils down to is plain and simple energy.

The DNA or genetic material of the strep determines its smell, color, form and characteristic shape; and when strep infects your tonsils or throat it is like the hair dryer that interferes with the television picture. A different energy with a different wavelength and different frequency is interfering with your own. The interference that shows up as static and glitches in a television is just like the interference in your energy. The symptoms with strep are pain or pus, but what is really happening is that your energy is being disrupted by the foreign energy of the germ.

Infection is simply a disruption in your natural energy patterns. This way of looking at germs can help you to increase your resistance to infection, and help you overcome infection more efficiently if you are already ill.

Disruptions of your energy can be prevented or reduced if you use other sources of energy more efficiently and work with the energy balancing mechanisms that are naturally available to you.

You take in energy to fuel and balance your system from sunshine, air, and food. Sound, climate and temperature, and chemical energy affect your energy as well. Releasing your pent-up energy (anger, grief, joy) through the safety valves of emotions is important, too. Maintenance of your energy, tuning it up and aligning it accounts for the importance of exercise and physical fitness.

When you understand disease as disrupted energy, you begin to appreciate health in a common sense way. You need energy to heal. You need your own energy to be strong so that foreign energies (which are present everywhere, all the time) will not interfere with your own.

Food has its own energy, and live food – food as it appears in nature, such as nuts, fruits, seeds, vegetables – is full of life energy. It takes much less of your own energy to digest an apple than a piece of bacon that is actually a slab of frozen, greasy, fried, preserved, *dead pig*. Not only that, but the apple actually *returns* life energy to you. All live foods impart an aliveness to you, a vital essence and vitality that cannot be measured in test tubes or quantified by counting calories or carbohydrates, proteins, vitamins or trace elements. The closer your food is to the way it was found in nature (uncooked, unprocessed, unrefined, not exposed to irradiation or chemicals, and not having passed through factories or packaging facilities), the more life energy is in it. When a food's molecules have not been tampered with the life energy in that food is available to and compatible with your own energy system. Heat, chemicals, irradiation, and other processing changes the molecular structure of your food. This makes the food's life energy less useful to you, *and* makes your system work hard, wasting its own energy to digest it. If food is what is alive and what gives us energy then junk food is a misnomer. It isn't food at all, but merely junk!

Calories are just a measure of the amount of heat that is generated in a test tube when a specific amount of a specific food is burned. *What happens in a test tube is just not the same as what happens in the body.* Calories were a useful concern in the past. Now however, because the food we eat is much more refined, processed, concentrated, dehydrated, radiated and medicated, a typical "calorically well-balanced" meal will have hundreds of preservatives, additives and chemicals, and just be more dead than alive. Caloric measurements are becoming outmoded. Healthful *available* energy for the body can just no longer be measured by counting calories, because the "food" that scientists burn to produce the heat is often not really food at all!

Smoke – from factories, cars, buses and cigarettes –is foreign energy that interferes with the natural energy you are taking in when you breathe. Air that is free of chemical pollutants keeps our own life energy in balance. Smoke's foreign energy disrupts our own — not just the energy of our lungs but the energy of our *entire* body.

Alcohol and drugs (whether they are illegal, prescribed, or over-the-counter) play havoc with our life energy. They drain and waste our energy, as every cell within us tries to cope with the out-of-sync condition they produce. Eventually, our cells come to mistake that condition for their natural state, and the drugs or alcohol become required to maintain that out of balance state. Withdrawing from addictions lets the body's energy return to its real, balanced, natural state.

Sometimes our own energy can build up beyond our capacity to use it. Emotions are energy. Just as pent-up energy in a car's motor can blow rods and radiators, so pent-up emotional energy can blow holes in our stomachs, inflame our joints, induce back spasms, strokes, or even foster the development of cancer.

When we sit in air conditioned cars, homes and offices all summer, or when we live in stuffy, heated spaces all winter, we stress our natural energy. The constant, daily changes from warm to cold and cold to warm as we go outside and come inside, challenge our systems. Just as glass will break from an abrupt change from heat to cold or cold to heat, our cells, too, react with shock when we choose to live in overheated rooms instead of wearing an extra sweater when it's chilly. If we allowed our natural body thermostats to work unimpeded — if we would simply perspire more — we would be much more comfortable in the summer. Our energy *can* adjust to seasonal changes in temperature, but we burden it unnecessarily with abrupt, daily changes to "out of season" temperatures.

Once you understand infection and disease as disruptions in your natural energy, or interference by foreign energy, it is easy to see how natural temperatures, a quiet mind, unprocessed foods, an absence of caffeine, alcohol, nicotine and other chemical substances can help to keep you well. You begin to understand how to use the energy around you for health and healing.

You are surrounded all the time by trillions of viruses, mold, fungi and the types of energy patterns or distinctive light waves we call germs. (There are more germs naturally on us and in us than we have cells, and we have trillions of cells!) Isn't it amazing that so very few people actually *do* become infected with strep, cold viruses, meningitis or flu "bugs" when trillions of those germs are on us or in us, or both?! (Even when "the flu is going around," and it seems as if everyone has it, more people actually don't have it than do. They're just less conspicuous because they aren't sniffling or coughing or absent from work.)

Despite the foreign energy present in your energy field – all the germs living quietly on your tonsils, for example – you usually stay well. Just like a television screen showing a perfect picture while hundreds of hair dryers, electric shavers, heating pads and microwave ovens operate in the same apartment building, your body can function amid lots of potential disruptions.

Your energy system generally has sufficient resistance to foreign energy frequencies, vibrations and wavelengths, such as germs, to stay in balance and remain well, *if you live a healthy lifestyle. Otherwise not!* The mechanism within your system that balances, resists and compensates for the presence of foreign energy is homeostasis. It is your healing force, your own set of fine tuning controls that keep your vertical and horizontal holds, your brightness and contrast, and your focus working just right!

When you are well, your body is resonating on a healthful, balanced frequency and wavelengh. Strep and other germs can live in your mouth by the billions without causing disruption until something disturbs your body's energy pattern. When your resistance to energy interference decreases, the strep frequency is able to intrude. Where a television screen would show static, you develop fever and pain when you swallow. Your homeostatic force is overcome by a foreign energy and you have tonsillitis or a strep throat or the flu.

There are several paths on which infection can travel. Disruption of your energy which allows for infection can occur through exposure to a particularly virulent germ whose energy is powerful enough to overcome most resistance. There are really very few of these that have ever been around. Most people do not get meningitis even when living in an

Army barracks infested with the germ. Most people don't get the flu when it is epidemic, and most people did not get the plague when it raged during the Middle Ages.

Infection can also occur when various germs find their way into places in your body where they just don't belong. It is comparable to touching a hot, electrically live bare wire to the transistors in a television set. The set will blow. In your system, gonorrheal germs emit a frequency that is not tolerable to the mucous membranes of the eyes, throat, rectum, penis, or vagina. Gonorrheal energy will more times than not disrupt normal surrounding mucous membrane energy and cause disease.

The AIDS virus is an example of energy gaining a stronghold in locations where it disrupts surrounding energy. The virus has undoubtedly been with us for a long time, but its virulence emerged only after it settled in mucous linings of the rectum, or in linings of the veins of drug users or patients receiving contaminated transfusions. There it exerts its disruptive energy force.

Western medicine may be backwards in the way it deals with infection. An infection such as strep may not occur because the tonsils are invaded with strep. That theory may be no more correct than the not-too-old theory that maggots cause flesh to rot. It took centuries to discover that it is the rotting flesh that allows maggots to grow and flourish. So it may be with most infections. When tonsil or throat energy is disrupted, *then* the streptococcus germ, which has been living there all along, can begin to grow and flourish.

Our treatment of strep infection is not very smart! We spend a great deal of time and money culturing the throat and killing the strep with the energy that Penicillin emits. We use the Penicillin to treat the pus, the pain, the fever and to prevent a secondary energy imbalance called rheumatic fever. This treatment is the equivalent of cleaning the maggots off a slab of meat without addressing the factors that caused the meat to rot!

Our treatment causes as many problems as it solves. But this is because we have been stuck at the cellular level of thinking. We must get beyond that and witness our health at the energy level.

Our tonsils, ears, glands, intestines, kidneys, bladder and eyes become infected – their energy is disrupted – when they happen to become the point of least resistance in our entire systems. Other points of least resistance allow the development of backaches, hemorrhoids, and migraines.

The points of least resistance in your body are determined by your genes, your age, and your lifestyle. You have certain target organs for the physical, emotional and mental stresses your body experiences. Those are the organs most likely to have their energy disrupted and support the growth of your germs.

Allergy is foreign energy (molds, pollen, certain foods) that disrupts human energy and results in a physical reaction. Sneezing, coughing, asthma, gastrointestinal distress are simply evidence of energy disruptions; *more glitches in the "TV screen.''*

Addiction is the disruption of human energy through the unhealthful incorporation of a foreign energy. Your energy fields wind up actually requiring the foreign energy for "pseudobalance," and you become ill (your energy is disrupted) when the substance is not present. This process is witnessed clearly through well-known withdrawal symptoms. Whether you are giving up alcohol, tobacco, narcotics or even caffeine (for which a special caffeine-withdrawal headache has been identified), your withdrawal symptoms are the result of your body's energy not accepting the absence of the foreign energy to which it had become accustomed. When a real balance is restored, the addiction is over, and health may resume.

I have observed in my practice that a craving for or an "addiction" to certain foods may indicate an allergy to that food. Because allergic reactions involve the subversion of the body's immune system, once the subversion takes place, a new balance or "pseudobalance" occurs. The new balance, to maintain itself, requires the original allergy-causing substance.

In the classic allergy reaction, the body's energy short-circuits in the spasm reaction. In the case of addiction, we take in foreign energy, the body incorporates the foreign energy into its own circuits and realigns itself to a different wavelength of energy. The trouble is that this new wavelength is ultimately destructive to the entire system.

From whatever source it comes – air molds, pills, junk that passes for food, germs – we need to understand that foreign energy is foreign energy. This energy model of disease (dis-ease) will enable us to get well and stay well by addressing energy imbalance. We will know how to go back to our innate, natural, personal, correct, individualized main source of energy. By increasing our body's resistance to foreign energy we will be able to keep the body well. And by cleaning up our environment, both inside and outside the body, we will achieve the highest level of *Wellness*.

Chapter Six

I Lack Love
(I-L-L)

In these times of loosening family bonds and heightened levels of stress, the natural separation process that occurs between a mother and child between six months and three years after birth is interpreted by the child as abandonment. Children's feelings of abandonment throughout childhood are especially keen. A child views the world with himself at its center, so feelings of abandonment program thoughts of unworthiness. These thoughts, programmed so early in life, manifest themselves throughout the person's life. They often become a cry for attention in the form of illness.

In this context, I like to think of ill as an acronym for I Lack Love.

Freud, Jung, Adler and others assessed the results of the "I Lack Love" imprinting, but misinterpreted the cause. They then built complex explanations of human behavior that generally are not helpful because they miss the point. The point is that *to the developing or maturing person, the feelings of love or lack of love determine future action, behavior and thought.* All other explanations are essentially the result of scientifically sophisticated minds trying as best they can to explain the workings of the mind.

Imprinted in all of us since early childhood is a filter through which we see the world. The filter alters the lens through which we evaluate, judge, and deal with life. We can see everything through the harsh expectations of our parents, with memories of their drug or alcohol or physical abuses, unreliability, or insensitivity. Or exactly the opposite if that was the case. These filters are imprinted during every childhood experience. If we grew up watching *Ozzie and Harriet* or *Father Knows Best,* or admiring Norman Rockwell's paintings, we developed certain expectations that tinted our filters. When we see our lives through those filters and judge our performance in life through those expectations, we can live our entire lives feeling as if something is not measuring up. This feeling is stressful, and can lead to continual states of dis-ease.

After childhood, there is the filter of "I Lack Love" through which we view all of our subsequent existence. But we can diminish, neutralize and even extinguish the energy that enables the "I Lack Love" programming to exist.

We misunderstand love in Western society. We believe that it is bestowed by others upon us, when, in fact, a different model works much better. The basic life energy I have been writing about throughout this book is the real love that exists in abundance in every living thing. It is within us, it is self-replenishing, and we only have to recognize its presence within us in order to reap its rewards. All the great spiritual leaders in history and in all the world religions spoke of this love. The energy with which this love resonates is the most powerful energy there is. This energy is special in that the more of it we share with others, the more of it comes back to us. You can't run out of it, and it can't be taken away from you. The world resonates with it, and we resonate with it. It is the nature of love to make itself more available the more it is shared, spread around and celebrated.

We never have to blame any one else for love's absence in our lives, because it is never absent! When someone loves us in the Western way of thinking, what they are really doing is letting the love that's inside us all the time come to the surface. When we are heartbroken or bereaved, our feelings of abandonment are legitimate, but there is no less love in our lives. The catalyst for our recognizing love may go away, but the love is inside us all the time.

The good news, even for skeptics, is that we *can* learn to tap into this love and reap its rewards, no matter how old we are, no matter how unloved we may feel! It is never too late to find the healing love that's inside us all.

John Andrews, a patient of mine, was *eighty six years old* when he first discovered how his early childhood programming was keeping him sick. A dramatic change took place when he found the source of his energy – his love – and let the healing process begin.

John has come into my clinic for a sixty minute consultation with Serina Taub, a health facilitator

*and registered nurse. His statements are excerpted
below. John begins:*

"I'm not ready to die. . .

"I've had a terrible accident.

"I'd been a university professor for fifty years.
I'm eighty-six years old now. All my friends
when they retired didn't do anything; they just
got arthritis and things and they just stopped. I
think there's more to life than that. I'm so
restless. Now I review concerts for newspapers.
I've also written fifteen hundred musical pieces
and gotten second place awards in national
competitions since I retired.

"I'm so confused now. I need everything done
for me. I need help so much. I had a terrible
accident. Six months ago I was riding a bus
crowded with kids coming home from the
beach. Oh! It was so terrible. Two teenage
boys kicked me through the door at a bus stop.
It was so terrible; I had a heart attack from the
shock. I felt so bad that after all the good work
I've done for people that kids would act like
that.

"They put me in the hospital for two weeks,
and I felt it was too long, and no one ever really
asked me about what my feelings were or about
my philosophy or what I want to do. All they

did was pump more and more medicines into me. Oh! I'm taking seventeen different bottles of medicines now and I just can't take it any more. Now they want to add more Lasix, and something inside me says it isn't the way.

"I'm not ready to die. It's a disgrace. I need help so much. I feel I can get away from some of the medicines and start taking natural things. I'm just getting toxic reactions; I can't speak right. I can't remember things. I can't even think — and all the medicine isn't even lowering my blood pressure.

"I've got four physicians and I know I need some medicines, but not seventeen of them. I don't even know what they are or what they are for. I'm not even sure what this 'heart shock' is, that the doctors said I have. They won't tell me. They won't even tell me what the drugs are for.

"My doctors are harassing me to come back for medicine, but they are only interested in appearances; they refuse to ask me about my philosophy or what I'm about or what I even think. I meditate now. I did it in the hospital and the nurses were so scared that something was wrong, because I was so quiet.

"When I came to California I was one of the first persons to challenge the fact that people

over sixty-five shouldn't be allowed to teach. I
sent all my degrees and credentials to the state
and I now have a certificate to teach. I taught
history for fifty years in New York and
California."

*(The nurse poses a question here: "What is your
life's purpose?")*

"My life's purpose is to help people. But I
haven't been able to do it for myself. I feel like I
have this inner tension that prevents me from
doing things. I have this whole array of
potentials, but I feel shaky and unstable.
Actually I've never had a well day in my life.
I've never been without a medicine for one
disease or another.

"I have so much water in me now. I have sixty
extra pounds of water in me. My toes are so
swollen I can't move them. I'm on a very strict
low-sodium diet. I have no physical restrictions,
but the weight increase won't let me do
anything. The swelling began five weeks ago,
and now my breathing is difficult and labored. I
don't feel right about the medicines I'm on.

"This medical care is so confusing to me. I've
had to change doctors so many times and their
fees are so high; thirty dollars for a blood
pressure test is too much. I can't understand
why my doctors won't let me drink water; every

one of my doctors won't let me drink water. I'm so fed up with the diuretic pills I take four times a day and all I'm allowed is a small cup of tea each day and I don't know if these doctors are right and I don't know what to do but I think I need to drink more water.

"I'm trying to eat as much fresh fruit as possible and I don't take alcohol. I have some jam and some sugar cubes for energy. I urinate six or eight times a day and I can't understand why I'm still so bloated. I wish I had just one doctor. One who would take the whole me into account, but I don't know how to do the research to find one. I need to do something because I can't even get my four doctors to pay attention to what the others are giving me."

(The nurse suggests that he take a twenty minute walk each day and find a single doctor.)

"Ok, I'll walk everyday. I'd rather go to one doctor, but as soon as they get me they throw me in the hospital and that's it. They all send for my records and then when Medicare bills me they want me to get three more opinions on what's going on with me and I think that means I'm supposed to go see even more doctors. I don't know where to go or what to do. It would be so marvelous if I only knew who to listen to. I'm going to listen; my mind is willing and my

heart is willing, but I've got to understand what
to do.

"Last week, the water in me just rolled into my
scrotum. I'm so embarrassed and uncomfortable.
I'm bigger than two grapefruits in my scrotum
now. . ."

*(The rest of John's story poured out of him after the
nurse led him through a healing meditation
designed to unleash his own healing forces, set
goals, and get inspiration.)*

"Why did this accident happen and what does
it mean to me and why does it seem to be
impairing me for life? Why is it all hanging on
so long? I feel I'm a very angry person but it's
not doing me any good.

"Now I know why I'm angry. It's because I've
been so crucial to students. By helping them all
my life. And they advance. Presidents, vice
presidents. Major companies. Such successes.
I'm angry that they've all advanced and I'm
just in the doldrums, and all I do is just go on
and on and I have nothing for it. I keep looking
at the material rewards that others receive."

*(The nurse comments that John seems to be
lacking in spiritual values and that he judges
himself and doesn't appear to like himself very
much. She says that she understands John doesn't*

want to die yet and how strongly he feels that he is not ready to die yet. She suggests it's time to reach the point in his life where he approves of himself).

"I've lived all my life wanting approval. I came from a really large family. My older brother was the patriarch and I had to work to support him through school and support the rest of the family. I gave and I gave and I gave. All my life I've given and given, but now for the first time I'm realizing that I've done it grudgingly. I've done it so grudgingly that I never felt I've been a good person. Even my mother said to me one day that I'd done enough, but I still felt obliged.

"Nurse, you say it's time to review my life. Okay, I've done these things and what I did was good. But my gift had a price tag; I needed to feel and be appreciated. I've learned from it though. I can at least give myself credit even though what I did for my family was out of guilt. You say that I needed the experience to learn how to say 'no' when I can't give anymore. That sometimes it's not helping a person to do for them. That now I must give to my own inner self. You're saying I've learned things and it's what I can take with me from the lifetime. Cherish my lessons.

"I've never helped others willingly. I'm shocked to realize that. I see it so clearly now.

But I can believe everything that is past is past, and I'm going to take those instances and pass on by; it all had meaning.

"All the events bringing happiness or sorrow have had meaning to me. I'm working on accepting myself before I pass on and I'm rebelling. I don't want to die before I'm clear. I've never found my inner self, and I purposely seem to find doctors who are just looking for what they can see. I myself just haven't been ready for someone to see the spiritual side of me.

"The accident is obviously a focal point for me now. It was a slap in my face. So what, that those kids did those things to me? So what, that that's why I'm angry? So what that I can't let it go. I've hurt myself so much because of my anger. Even though I'm a good person I haven't been able to accept it so far. I get loads of fan mail from my columns, and thank you notes every week from my students, but I'm discovering that it's never enough. It's got to come from within. I've judged myself so severely that now I'm dependent on society. I'm helpless. If I've never accepted myself how could I accept others? I've put up this mask about all that I've done for humanity, but inside I've just never felt I'm good. I said, 'Oh, I must give to prove to myself that I'm good.'

"I've been touched greatly by this office visit
and by the meditation and your kindness and
caring. I've never delved into myself as deeply;
all I have done is get angry. I've always been
searching through poetry and drama and all the
other things. I'm at the point where I need to
make peace with myself . . . **Oh my God, *my
toes are beginning to move!* The water is
leaving my toes** . . . where is the washroom?
This has been a wonderful revelation for
me. . . "

*(John leaves for the restroom and experiences a
remarkable instantaneous diuresis (large amount of
urine and loss of body fluids) and then says, in a
whisper:)*

"Now this is what I finally understand. This is
what I'll tell you. My father was a Norwegian
and he married an Indian girl. That came out in
elementary school and they called me all sorts
of terrible and violent names. *I made up my
mind years ago that I'd never love anybody.*

"I've been trying to protect myself. Now
you've helped me go so deep within myself that
I just know I can survive. . . *I can even forgive
my parents for loving each other so much in
spite of what society thought.* This has been
with me all my life. Every person has their own
cross to bear and I've never learned to accept
mine. Even when all the kids called me names I

tried to protect myself. I wrote a poem once
about *I don't even know what race I am.* I
have been laboring under this thing for all these
years. I never loved anyone. I have just never
loved anyone. I never loved myself. I never
married. But I'm not too old though. . . *Isn't
this wonderful? Isn't this wonderful?*

"I've been angry all my life because I was born
who I was. I've lacked love and I've never
forgiven myself."

John's remarkable story speaks for itself; he
went on to lose forty pounds of water in the next
five weeks and actually became *well* enough to
begin dating a lovely lady that was his own age. But
let's just review a few of the circumstances he
reveals as he comes to face the "I Lack Love"
condition. He is obviously a talented and energetic
man. Yet his own early life didn't give him the
advantage of the good start he probably deserved.
Instead he had to subjugate his own life to his
brother's. He has spent the rest of his life resenting
the "head start" he has given to all those students
who went on to become top executives.

The crowning blow is when the kids on the bus –
kids like the very ones he has done so much for –
literally give him a slap in the face, as he says, or a
kick in the pants.

It almost kills him, but John is a strong and
stubborn individual (or he would never have gotten
this far). He is able, when the chips are down, to find

the help he needs to find himself. In the beginning, notice the words he uses. He doesn't say, "I was mugged by a bunch of hoodlums," or "Teenage thugs attacked me." He has so given himself over to the victim mentality that he actually describes the *attack* as an *accident*; as if it were nobody's fault except possibly his own.

But John does not want to die. He makes remarkably quick use of the simple healing meditation we offered him, and in a single session comes to terms with the deep roots of his anger. In the beginning he couldn't mention it. He couldn't get back any farther than a passing mention of his brother. Only at the end can he talk about his parents and the abandonment he felt at their having brought him into a world where from the beginning he could find no place for himself, no tribe of people to belong to. He felt truly outcast from his earliest memories, but he is a determined man. An optimist! Even at eighty-six he says maybe it's not to late to get married! In any case, it is not too late for John to love himself. A remarkable man.

When connectedness (in terms of energy, a natural bonding) has been suppressed or repressed; when you feel apart from the rest of humanity, the result is disastrous to spirit, mind and body as it hinders the development of self-esteem. In John's case there was a lack of bonding not only to individuals, but to the whole human race. His case was an extreme one, but it is the rare individual who comes to adulthood unscathed. People who are lonely, especially older people, too often feel separate from other people. Often they use their diseases as a topic of conversation to make contact with others! We all need to learn to foster our self-esteem. Self-esteem is vital to establish *Wellness*. The most powerful builder of self-esteem is to love and be loved.

What are some of our own thoughts about yourself? Do you think you are unworthy? Do you value yourself? Do you think you are a failure for not having lived up to your own or others' expectations? Do you feel guilty? Do you lack enough love for yourself to forget about seat belts, keep on smoking or drinking, get colds, migraines, backaches and lapse into hidden levels of despair that lead to illness?

You are continuously being bombarded and assaulted with messages and reminders of war, holocaust, hijacking, rape, sodomy, AIDs, nuclear accidents, battered children, terrorism, murder, disease, filth, perversion. These negative images are the last things in your mind as you watch the evening news before your so-called "night of rest." The continuous negativity separates your mind from the beauty of life, and the love of God that elevates your value and esteem in yourself. It is almost as if dark forces have taken over to separate you and your thoughts from the consciousness or the memory of a loving and Supreme Being. It is no wonder then that I-L-L has become equivalent to *I Lack Love.*

Chapter Seven

"The Thinker"

BE HAPPY NOT RIGHT

Be happy: it is more important than being right. Whatever erroneous beliefs and thoughts are programmed into your mind will start to surface as you get closer to getting on the bridge to *Wellness*. The five-week program removes the milestone of incorrect programming from around your neck and unsticks you from the muck and mire of your thoughts, attitudes, convictions and beliefs that are keeping you sick and tired.

It is so difficult to get well for so many people because you have to process the healing ideas through the very thoughts, the very belief system and ego that are causing the problem in the first place. And your ego is very comfortable where it is, or it wouldn't be there. The fact that you are not comfortable, that you are dis-eased, doesn't influence your ego at all.

Until you cross the bridge to *Wellness* and look at your thoughts from the viewpoint of the other side, it is difficult to believe that your illnesses and lack of energy begin in your mind, and that the way out of the muck and mire where you are stuck lies in changing your mind and correcting the erroneous thoughts that cause your difficulties.

These are the kinds of erroneous thoughts that are keeping us from *Wellness*:

- That arthritis is chronic.
- That cancer is fatal.
- That schizophrenia is for life.
- That calories are the key to slimness.
- That milk makes you healthy.
- That red meat is good for you.
- That grown men don't cry.
- That kids wet the bed because they're sound sleepers.
- That eyesight can't improve.
- That older age is associated with flagging sexual drive.
- That it is normal for kids to have headaches and diarrhea, tonsillitis or bronchitis, flu or rashes or earaches or any other illness a few times a year.
- That boys need to be circumcised.
- That children need to be delivered by Caesarean section.
- That you need to have your uterus removed for bleeding or your breasts irradiated with yearly mammograms, or your body stress-tested and cardiographed and prodded in yearly physicals to stay well.

- That risking openness in relationships leads to tragedy, or that faith is for the uneducated or that love hurts.
- That you catch cold for no reason.
- That too much fruit is not good for you or that you should not eat too many avocados.
- That you suffer backaches, migraines, stomach problems, hypertension and gout because it is your lot in life to do so.
- That medicine is the best remedy for hypertension.
- That once you have insulin-dependent diabetes you are stuck with injections forever.

Do you believe you have a *"bad"* back, or *"weak"* lungs, or a *"sensitive"* stomach? Do you *"think"* you don't have time to exercise or that you *"can't"* lose weight or stop smoking? Do you *"think"* you are *allergic, sickly* or *need* a drink of alcohol?

Here are a few examples of thoughts that block our inner healing forces that surfaced in only one typical morning of patient care:

Dan Rivers, a 52-year old executive, told me he *"caught"* cold from working out at his club, perspiring and then "stupidly lying down on the cold floor to rest for a minute" . . . and then began sneezing and *"knew"* the cold was coming on. As I asked him when he first heard that getting cold while perspiring causes colds, I thought of the millions of Scandinavians and thousands of skiers who go from hot springs or Jacuzzis to cold romps in the snow, or from saunas to cool showers.

Dan said his parents drummed the thought into his head ever since he could remember, that getting chilled while perspiring meant instant sickness and problems. You didn't do that in his household. He recollected his mortification at being the only kid in his Boston Irish neighborhood who had to wear galoshes just to play in the dewy grass if the day was cold.

Louise Miller is a 34-year old draftswoman who came to see me because of a year-long backache that was not responding to chiropractic treatment, rest, traction or anti-inflammatory and muscle-relaxant medication. She proceeded to let me know rather directly, three times in our first session, that "drafting was no good for the back."

As Louise and I began to discuss her belief about drafting and its "badness" for the back, it became clear that she was desperately seeking strength to get out of her field, leave her job and go back to college where she could begin meeting people and eventually form a meaningful relationship. She needed to overcome the intense loneliness she had been experiencing over the years. She was hunched over the drafting table in a no-nonsense office of other women, with an utter lack of contact, closeness or merriment of any kind. Her belief was an effective yet physically painful way of forcing a decision on herself to quit her occupation, a decision that she was otherwise unable to make.

I asked Louise where she first heard that drafting was bad for the back and she recalled her mother telling her as early as the first grade that if she didn't sit up straight at school and at home doing her handwriting and drawing she would absolutely have a bad back and that was that. And Louise could only do her drafting well if she was hunched over.

Susan Rivers, a 13-year old, came to see me because she had experienced menarche, her first menstrual period. Susan's mother proceeded to tell me in front of her daughter that Susan now had the same severe menstrual cramping all the women in the family have, including herself, and her other two daughters. Mother wanted some medication, perhaps birth control pills for hormonal effects, so that Susan could avoid, she went on to say, the chronic problem "that would bother her the rest of her life."

The examples go on and on, but what it boils down to is that you have been taught to think special thoughts in special ways that are not healthful. Then you are blocked from thinking your way out of the thought or belief because of the mental programs you are stuck with. These thoughts begin with "I Lack Love" and continue because of the "S Factor".

Even in my own life I have seen how the thoughts programmed into my mind from a very young age have affected my health as an adult. Until seven years ago, I would catch a cold immediately if I got caught in the rain, felt my hair get wet, or got slightly chilled. My grandmother always warned me that getting caught in the rain without a hat was inviting pneumonia or "at the very least a cold."

Three years ago I developed pneumonia after "getting caught" (in my own yard, and in a warm, California, not a cold, New York, rain). As my hair got wet and I began to sneeze, for just a millisecond there was the clear vision–deja vu–of Grandma saying, *"Eddie boy, button your coat and put on your hat so your hair doesn't get wet and you catch a cold or pneumonia."* Well, this time the California heat and the fact that the cold progressed to pneumonia and the fact that the sneezing started at the moment my hair got wet, opened what seemed like a giant steel door in my mind and I felt as if a claw were binding me down to a thought, a conviction that was able to make me sick. I became instantly aware that the thought was wrong and unheathful. By that sheer awareness I was able to grapple with the notion, look at it, remove the claw, and come to the clear determination that it would never do me in again. And it doesn't. And it won't. How do I know? The same way I know I will never smoke again after quitting a 25-year habit more than seven years ago. The same way I know I won't wet the bed again as I did 40 years ago; a habit that persisted for 10 years because of inner tension and stress, while the doctor reassured everyone that I was just a deep sleeper.

As you approach *Wellness*, as you begin to cross the bridge from sick and tired to *Wellness*, a new awareness will develop. That awareness will occur at a deep, inner level. It occurs and never leaves. It's like learning to ride a bicycle or how to make love or what an apple tastes like. When you discover this awareness of your personally detrimental thoughts or behaviors, the awareness itself will automatically lead to changes *if you have a will to live and a high regard for or reverence for life.*

Your voyage to *Wellness* is going to generate reverence and the "will to be well." *That's what the Prescription For Life is all about.* The meditation and exercise especially, but really every ingredient of the Prescription For Life will help establish new circuits and connections in your brain. You will establish new patterns of expectation, beliefs, and behavior that will reprogram yourself into *Wellness.*

Americans are the most obese, hypertensive, atherosclerotic, gouty, ulcer-ridden, arthritic, cancer and coronary prone population in the world. We are the most over medicated, over radiated, over surgerized people since the beginning of recorded history — because of what we *think!* Now it is more important to be happy rather than right!

Your old, destructive thoughts and beliefs will be supplanted with new chemical and nervous system pathways. New possibilities for new health will result from new beliefs and new behaviors. Good health becomes as inevitable as gravity once the awareness is there. Old habits, appetites and illness producing thoughts and ideas are replaced with their opposites. *Wellness* is natural and inevitable when your awareness meets the full force of your life energy.

CAUTION: EGO AT WORK –

There are many choices for you to be healthy and well: books and breakthroughs in nutrition, exercise, attitude and communication. There are options that excite you and lead you to follow new, sensible programs with confidence and enthusiasm. Yet time after time you fall off the wagon without knowing what has happened (something I will discuss more in "The Last Hurdle").

You wind up where you started because you are doing too well! No matter how good your intentions are, your ego, which is a composite of all your beliefs, thoughts, prejudices, hopes, fears, attitudes and convictions, *will do anything to survive in the state that it is in.* When you do well and threaten to change it, your ego backs you off your path before you get a chance to alter the thoughts that make it up.

Make no mistake about the power of your ego. It makes diabetics continue to smoke as their legs are being amputated for small-vessel, nicotine-induced disease. It makes people jump out of windows rather than apologize or settle a feud. It reverts to absolute psychosis – makes you "crazy" if that is what's necessary for the ego to defend itself. You are often in a trap, a road without an exit. The bridge to *Wellness* offers you a way to change direction.

Not only is your own ego always on the lookout for threats to it, but others in your lives have *their* egos watching out for change as well. The role of caretaker in your life, whether played by your mother, your wife or husband, even your child or doctor, is protected by that person's ego! If *you* get well, you change that person's role. That person's ego fights change – even changes in *your* life – because egos are very tenacious! That is why, without knowing it, many people really help each other to stay sick, overweight, addicted or run down. A change in your health would require a change in others' roles in your life, and their egos will fight to keep things the way they are!

One of my patients was a man confined to a wheelchair. He had multiple sclerosis and owned a grocery store. His wife took very good care of him. After he was meditating and following this program, he felt better about himself than ever before. His dependence on his wife for physical assistance lessened a great deal, and he opened three new grocery stores. He also began telling everyone he knew about how the meditation was helping him. Well, his wife was very threatened by this change in her husband's life. She felt unneeded as his need to be taken care of decreased. She was embarrassed by his giving credit to meditation, as if she were jealous that she never got that kind of praise and attention for taking such good care of him over the years. They argued a lot and the tension between them increased as their new roles in the relationship were developing.

If you are sensitive to the needs and egos of the other people in your life, you will be able to make positive choices for your health with their support.

If they cannot straight-out support you, at least they will allow you your new behaviors and new health. Just be aware that the ego, yours and your family's is a strong, defensive fighter for the status quo!

The most powerful way that your ego—the *collection of all your thoughts, attitudes, impressions and opinions* — has to defend itself and to literally prevent its death, is through what I call the *"Thinker."* Your *"Thinker"* is comprised of all the thoughts you have ever had from all of the books you have read, the movies you have seen the stories you have heard and the events you have experienced.

In this day and age of stress your *"Thinker"* takes on a strength and power which is just about unlimited in its ability to cause you to worry and fear and expect illness and enslave you to your ego. Your *"Thinker"* has been programmed with powerful disease-ridden advertisements, violent newscasts, reports of molested, tortured and missing children, holocaust, rape, hijacking, war, etc., etc. Your *"Thinker"* becomes virtually autonomous and independent and constantly attacks your peace of mind.

You *think* that good nutrition is a bore, that exercise is too time consuming, that cigarettes are necessary and that another cocktail will make you feel better. Your *"Thinker"* is the reason you need a prescription or a bridge—*a strategy*—to get from sick and tired to healthy and well. *You certainly can't use the same thoughts that are causing your problems in the first place to eliminate your problems.*

MEDIA AND WORLD VIEW:
HOW OUR GREAT-GRANDPARENTS'
WORLD WAS DIFFERENT

There are so many more illness-inducing influences, and so much more stress today than during the time our great grandfathers were splitting logs and struggling to keep the home fires burning. The breakup of the old-fashioned family and the nurturing bonds of the extended family are major reasons why we feel more stress today. The support systems humans have depended on through history for nurture and nourishment are collapsing under the weight of modern life, with its high technology, high divorce rate and the incessant distractions provided by the media.

A vivid example of the media's influence on our minds and its resultant stress could be seen on a recent NFL/AFL playoff day. Tens of millions of people, their attention riveted on the football game, saw an advertisement for a movie to be shown later on the same channel. Minds and thoughts froze on the image of the terror about to engulf the happy family of a doctor . . . a shining knife is raised, and laughs of happy children turn to screams of terror as daddy or someone cuts mommy and them to pieces. This kind of intrusion into our homes, our minds, our eyes and ears not only can cause illness –a headache beginning, a back spasm, blood pressure climbing – but further weakens the image of family bonds that are already weakening too fast in our society.

Great-grandfather just didn't have the constant mind-rape we experience even while trying to enjoy the good old American classic, Sunday football. He didn't have traffic, smog, insecticides, acid rain, radiation, wide-scale pornography, the holocaust and the ugly rest. Of course the world wasn't perfect. There were wars, economic hardships, natural disasters and man's inhumanity to man.

But there were major differences between the stress of those events and today's. He viewed the world through a conviction that God loved and would take care of his family and his country; that he loved and was loved by his family, that he had a place in his family, his community and his country. His conviction, his attitude, was spelled out continuously in a stream of literature from DeTocqueville to Steinbeck. We may regard that conviction as simplistic and old-fashioned, but please notice it revolved around a center of faith and love, those crucial elements to human well-being. That conviction and the frame of mind it brought are what alleviated and dissipated the stress that now drives his grandchildren to mental despair and physical deterioration.

In order to be well, we must be prepared to outdistance the blockers of *Wellness*. We may help ourselves by keeping our great-grandparents' example in front of us. Love, laughter, hope and faith lead us at last to the Prescription For Life.

STRESS AND DISEASE

Stress has become the new national virus. It underlies virtually all our diseases. Stress—*physical, mental, emotional and spiritual*—occurs because of how we think and the *thoughts* that we think with —particularly thoughts that lead to unhealthy lifestyles, detrimental habits and behavior.

You have succumbed to stress when you cannot concentrate on anything for very long because your thoughts keep thinking—or when you *have* to smoke, drink or use drugs, or when you have caught cold, developed a backache, migraine, high blood pressure, ulcers, arthritis, diabetis and even cancer.

Stress comes from what you think, what you eat, what you breathe, what you hear, what you see, what you smell and what you touch.

Events, circumstances and people do not cause stress. It is our response and our appraisal of our ability to cope that causes stress.

If you cannot eliminate your boss and how he acts, you can still respond differently; if you can't stop the smog or the insectides that pollute you, you can still enhance your resistance to it. If you cannot eliminate traffic, car horns, prolonged wastes of time and angry drivers, you can change your response and reaction to it. If you cannot avoid photographs of battered children, chemical warfare, self-immolation and executed hostages, or news about holocaust, hijackings, aids, anal sex, acid rain, the greenhouse affect, teenage suicide, people going insane—you can still change your reaction and response to this too. *Stress begins between your ears*! Recently I witnessed a bicyclist, assumedly out for a nice afternoon ride, chase down and spit in the face of an elderly lady driving through supposedly peaceful Marin County, California—because her driving style slowed his frenetic pace!

Almost one third of American babies start life with a shocking interruption of their natural solitude; a Caesarean section, a rather dramatic and bloody procedure delivers them rapidly through their mother's abdomen with a jolt! Almost all babies are delivered into the intense glare of operating room lamps to be spanked and have tubes shoved down their noses, through their mouths and up their rectums. Almost half of American babies are circumcised in cold assembly-line fashion *without* anaesthetic; three quarters of our babies are fed refined, processed, lifeless formula; they are all temporarily blinded by a chemical that is instilled into their eyes. *And this stress occurs before young Americans even leave the hospital!*

Once home, American babies are exposed to smoggy air, acid rain, insecticides and get smoked at in 20 million homes. They are given prescriptions containing alcohol, belladonna and barbituates to alleviate the colic they experience as a reflection of the stress they perceive in parents who are struggling to meet rent or mortgage payments and pay for the two thousand to ten thousand dollar hospital bill that it costs just to be born!

By the age of three of four, American children watch about 20,000 TV commercials a year and become infused with images and inducements to illness, disease, violence, war, lust and sex. By the time young Americans enter kindergarten, *now a college-preparatory course*, they are so "stressed-out" that ten percent are candidates for prescriptions for powerful drugs used to control hyperactivity in the classroom. Speaking of the "S Factor"!

It is very natural for your mind to resist these thoughts and say, "Aha! This doctor first says disease begins in our mind and now he claims our illness is caused by stress. Whatever happened to genes, germs and accidents!" No! Please read this carefully: *Virturally all illness begins in the mind and stress is causing most disease to occur PREMATURELY before its time.*

Your mind, in one way or another, controls *EVERYTHING* that goes on in your body—your hormones, your nervous system, your organs, your cellular reactions and your immune system. As already discussed when for one reason or another, the mind allows our natural defenses to weaken, the body can even develop cancer.

Certainly there are some instances of dis-ease that may not involve the mind at its onset—such as the trauma of an accident or being born with a genetic problem—but then, it all eventually *becomes* a function of the mind.

For instance, people with Downs Syndrome (which was formerly called Mongolism) can perform amazing feats of learning and self care—

if it is not ingrained in their minds by others that they are invalids.

Quadriplegia is an example of a dis-ease *caused* by an accident that subsequently *strongly involves the mind:* some quadriplegics vegetate and die as useless depressed hopeless human beings—others become artists, musicians, poets, even athletes! People are often exactly what they think they are.

Your thoughts determine the way you feel—and the way that you feel in large part determines whether you are healthy or not—*whether you get well quickly or whether you won't.*

A lack of love for yourself as well as a lack of love for others has a markedly corrosive affect on your health. *"ILL"* is equivalent to "I Lack Love"; not just in a romantic sense of course, although that will do it too!

Just think about it for a moment. Do you lack enough love for yourself that you continue to smoke knowing it causes cancer, or eat junk food knowing it detracts from your appearance and adds to your coronary risk? Do you deny yourself the few seconds it takes to fasten your seatbelt even though most auto-accident-caused deaths could be prevented by wearing seatbelts? Do you neglect exercising or forget to take at least a few minutes a day for quiet time or mediation or prayer? How much good care do you give to yourself?

The list can go on and on. The important issue is that persistence in unhealthy lifestyles and detrimental behaviors are a result of a lack of self love and esteem.

Health is determined by personal responsibility, self value, and high regard and reverence for life. This basic principle of Integrative Medicine provides the rationale for the Prescription For Life. This five-week commitment stimulates personal responsibility, enhances self value and develops high regard and reverence for life.

My patients sign a *"Wellness* Contract" to specify what they are willing to do for themselves. This is an abrupt way of facing one's own mortality. We continuously hear people say, "I'd be willing to do anything to be healthy and well." This then is a "fish or cut bait" confrontation – it helps one separate the wheat from the chaff; it is "personal responsibility time!"

For the next several chapters, this book will concentrate on the Wellness contract, highlighting each area.

Wellness is a state of mind and illness can be reversible by the power of your mind to heal. Following the Prescription For Life will absolutely enhance the quality of your life. There is also a significant probability of slowing down or reversing your disease and a real possibility of an absolute cure. You can now begin to control your health destiny by turning *"I Lack Love"* into *"I Love Life."*

Stress underlies virtually all of our diseases.

Cancer	Obesity	Aids
Stroke	Indigestion	Alzheimers
Ulcers	Asthma	Diabetes
Arthritis	Sexual Disorders	Psoriasis
Headaches	Accidents	Colds
Colitis	Depression	Backaches
Hypertension	Hemorrhoids	Coronary Disease
Impotency	Gout	Multiple Sclerosis

Stress is Spiritual:

Atonement	Isolation
Guilt	Hopelessness

Stress is Mental:

Worry	Anger	Lust
Fear	Resentment	Loneliness
Insecurity	Grief	Anxiety

Stress is Physical:

Alcohol	Radiation
Cigarettes	Insecticides
Drugs	Preservatives
Smog	Salt
Pollution	Refined Sugar
Acid Rain	Flourescent Lighting
Microwaves	Loud Sounds

Chapter Eight

Voyage to *Wellness*

Rx FOR LIFE

During my years in clinical medicine I began to notice, with increasing frequency, a phenomenon that had never been emphasized in my medical school training.

The phenomenon that I speak of is the relationship between health and thought. Year after year, I observed that families whose thoughts did not include the expectation of illness were almost never ill; while those who expected to be ill – very soon and very frequently –were. I called it the "80-20 phenomenon"; 20% of patients were ill 80% of the time. My clinical investigation of the "80-20 phenomenon" made me certain that a person's way of thinking and behaving played a major role in one's health – and that if certain thoughts, attitudes and behaviors could produce an unhealthy body, they could just as easily produce a healthy body!

These questions had to be answered. Accordingly, seven years ago, after making sure my patients were in good hands, I went on a sabbatical to study the relationship between physical health and thought, attitude and behavior. The pursuit of the answer has led me to over thirty nations and to the development of the Foundation for Health Awareness and the American Wellness Association.

While on this path of understanding I have met both men and women who have spent the greater parts of their lives looking deeply into the power of the mind and thought – not only as it affects our physical health, but how the very quality of our lives are in fact determined by the way that we think.

I no longer harbor any doubts about the results of how we think. We are, specifically in terms of our physical health, a mirror image of our personal thought processes. We are, in effect, the way we think we are.

Of course there are certain biological constraints and genetic limitations to take into account – the blind will not generally see nor the lame throw away their crutches – however, in general, illness in this age of stress begins in our mind and can be reversed through the power of the mind and the body to heal itself.

I now believe that I possess the single most effective tool to provide total health for my patients. It is the tool of understanding the power of thoughts, attitudes and feelings. **Patients can be taught to see for themselves how thought can produce illness. They can also be taught to reverse this power of thought to produce a totally healthy existence**.

My new practice of Integrative Medicine uses all the modern techniques of conventional medicine – drugs, surgery and radiation when absolutely necessary – however, the practice incorporates personal teaching and guidance in understanding how attitude, behavior and lifestyle lead to *Wellness* and health.

The *Wellness*-inducing tool my patients use is the Prescription For Life. It requires less than an hour a day of self-administered "TLC"! To really understand how the Prescription works, it is important to become aware of (or just review) a few of the concepts of Integrative Medicine.

There is a healing power residing in every single human cell. This awesome healing power is equivalent to the force that makes an acorn grow into an oak; this force is equivalent to the presence of God in every cell. If you want to be scientific, call it homeostasis or endorphins.

Our healing force is enhanced with live and vital food, honest and ethical behavior, prayer, faith, quiet times and meditation, sunshine and fresh air, lovingness, service to others, and safe behavior. Conversely, the healing force is blocked by barriers and dams we erect called worry, fear and anxiety; smoking, alcohol and drugs; dead, enbalmed, processed, denatured and unnatural foods; polluted air; radiation and unsafe behavior.

It is now time to suspend many of your assumptions about health and disease. What you have been taught and what you have taken for granted until now are not necessarily true.

Just as law doesn't always promote justice, a study of history does not prevent its repetition, and theology doesn't always lead to love of God, so Medicine does not always promote good health.

This is a time when enormous changes are

occurring in all fields. We are witnessing the most rapid advances of knowledge in recorded history. And Medicine is included. Only in the last decade has Medicine accepted that exercise can help reduce heart disease or that milk is not good for people with ulcers. By advancing your own thoughts in the field of Medicine you have a much better chance to get healthy and stay that way.

Now that you are familiar with the concepts of your mind's programming, anabolic life choices, templates, endorphins, the *smouldering stress syndrome* called the "S Factor" and life energy, it is time to lay down new neuronal and chemical pathways to extinguish the old and destructive ones that control your mind and body.

If you are a health-care professional or scientifically oriented, you can think of the bridge to *Wellness* that the Prescription For Life takes us across as a psychophysiological, self-reinforcing circuit. It takes five weeks to establish the curcuit in the mind and body. Most readers will be comfortable just thinking of it as a bridge from old thoughts to new ones.

Whoever you are, you can now be more certain than ever that you feel the way you think, and that virtually all disease begins in the mind. Taking care of your body is the best way to assure its taking care of you. The way you begin each day and look at the world – friendly or unfriendly, nurturing and supportive or negative and attacking – is a most significant factor in whether you stay ill or become well.

This *is* a Prescription. You *must* follow the directions. **To cross this bridge now requires your absolute attention. You must adhere strictly to the road signs and guideposts. You cannot make your own rules on this voyage because if you do, your old attitudes and thoughts will jump right in, and you will be thinking the very thoughts that caused you to need the Prescription For Life in the first place!**

After you read about the bridge, you will sign a health care agreement that will reinforce your willingness to be really well. You will give a copy of the agreement to your physician. You will also give a copy to someone else who will help you stay honest with yourself. Don't sign the agreement unless you are really ready to follow the Prescription and cross the bridge from being sick and tired. This Prescription *does* lead to *Wellness*, so you must be ready to accept *Wellness* before you start moving towards it!

There are seven sections to cross on the bridge to *Wellness*. Each section is an ingredient of the Prescription For Life. Crossing two or three or four sections cannot get you from here to there. You may feel slightly better; pretty good; almost well, yes; but really well and healthy, no! It is your choice, and it is now time to face it. Then confidently put your feet on the bridge and ignore the detours!

The seven sections on the bridge, ingredients of the Rx, are a quiet mind, exercise, nutrition, de-addiction, safety, lovingness and ethical behavior. Let's look at each of these more carefully.

INGREDIENT ONE: QUIETING THE MIND

The first section of the bridge is the most important and the easiest. It costs nothing and takes only twenty minutes a day. It can make you and other people very, very happy. This section of the bridge develops your sense of self-care and self-love and creates in you an attitude of increased self-worth and self-esteem.

Here is all you must do: every day for the next seven days, pick a time and sit down in a comfortable and quiet place where you will not be disturbed. Take the phone off the hook and tell your family not to disturb you for the next thirty minutes. You will practice meditation for about thirty minutes.

Meditation is the process of quieting the mind so thoughts stop. Endorphins flow, self healing begins, goal setting takes place and inspiration occurs. All this in just thirty minutes a day!

Meditation is more than relaxation or visual imagery. Both techniques are used as part of the meditation and are very useful, but they are not meditation. Meditation is fine-tuning and synchronizing the body, mind *and* soul. When the mind is still, the body can heal and the soul can be felt.

Some people say they commune with God during meditation. Others hear an inner voice or higher self. Still others experience a oneness with nature. The meditation experience is so difficult to describe because it is not measurable. It transcends rational, logical or sequential thought. What is the same for everyone, however, is that meditation does work to quiet the mind, stimulate the flow of healing endorphins, and make the mind hospitable to healing messages, positive goals, and inspiration. This process will help you become aware of your personal responsibility for your health and well being, and it will inspire you to move in that direction.

There are hundreds of meditation tapes, books, and methods available, but the special meditation therapy tape included with this book is especially suited for the specific changes you are about to make in your life. If you are already using transcendental meditation, structured prayer, or visualization every day, you may continue to do so. But listen to the Prescription For Life meditation therapy tape as well.* It is important that you include *three* key elements in your meditation, and this tape is designed with them in mind: *self healing, goal setting, and inspiration.*

This very simple thirty minute routine will put your brain in an alpha or theta rhythm (slow and calm), stimulate the flow of endorphins, replace unhealthy images in your mind with healthy ones, and give you inspiration about what you need to do to become healthy and well.

It is important that you suspend your need to agree or disagree when you listen to the meditation

*CAUTION: DO NOT LISTEN TO THE MEDITATION THERAPY TAPE WHILE YOU ARE DRIVING.

therapy tape. The reason this is important is that the relaxation/meditation process is directed to the right side of your brain, the side often described as creative, perceptive, intuitive, sensitive, imaginative. The side that takes over if you start agreeing or disagreeing is the analyzing, logical, deductive, quantifying left side of the brain. It's like trying to assess the beauty of the Mona Lisa using a computer. It might be an interesting exercise, but it's beside the point. So just go along with the voice on the tape and postpone or suspend your need to comment or critique the process during these few minutes.

If you insist on agreeing or disagreeing, know that it is only your ego—your *"Thinker"* struggling for survival. Each day that you follow the Prescription For Life, your *"Thinker"* weakens until it is overcome.

There are three parts to the meditation process on the Prescription For Life tape that comes with this book.

The *first* part of the meditation involves *breathing and self-healing* as you imagine a healing light moving through your body. This is the part that stimulates the flow of endorphins for healing. The endorphins will flow to the diseased heart, the swollen joints, the painful back and all the areas of the body in need of help – including the parts of the brain that are anxious and depressed.

The *second* part of the meditation involves *goal setting*. While your mind is deep in the meditative state you will paint on an imaginary canvas a mental picture of the way you want to look and feel. This is a very powerful part of the meditation because imagining is the very root of your power to be well. Imagining is actually at the root of all growth and creativity. Without imagining there would never have been a bridge built or a story written or a song composed. Change begins with an image in someone's mind!

The *third* part of the meditation involves *inspiration*. You will meet a guide or Master who will lead you toward change. You will learn of your own responsibility for your health and well being, and you will become more aware of your mission and the purpose of your life. You will reestablish the feeling of oneness with nature you experienced as a small child, lying in the grass, gazing at the stars on a balmy summer night.

As you meditate, you will do better and better each day. It is just like learning to drive or ski or swim. Every day you do it, it becomes more and more natural. Children and senior citizens seem to progress faster than people between those two groups. Older and younger people seem to imagine and pretend with more ease. Do not be discouraged if your mind doesn't quiet down. If you can't feel the light or hear the Master, it will all develop with time. After you meditate and reflect back on the experience, don't pay attention to the times your mind wasn't quiet. The important times are the moments when you just slip off and you are not thinking – even for only a few seconds – for *that* is when you are meditating!

Finally, just because your mind has been quiet and you have been unaware of your body, don't *think* you have been asleep! Meditation is a stage between wakefulness and sleep. When you open your eyes when the voice on the tape asks you to is evidence of your not having been asleep. In meditation you are actually super alert rather than asleep.

There will be times during the meditation when you will no longer be aware of the speaker's voice on the tape. That's wonderful! The tape is merely an aid. Do without it after a few weeks if you want to. You may find yourself meditating longer and longer each day. You will then feel more alert and refreshed as endorphins flow through your system unimpeded. If you do happen to fall asleep during the meditation (snoring, nodding off), that's okay too. Your healing endorphins will have been flowing during your rest. What a great way to get a healthy body! The point is, there is no way to "do it wrong!" Just do it every day and it will work for you!

Play the cassette and close your eyes. Breathe in exactly the manner explained on the cassette. After the guided meditation *write down* any notions that have come to you about the responsibility you need to take to be more healthy and well than you presently are. It's that simple.

During the meditation, thoughts and feelings will occasionally surface. Deal with these immediately. *There are three ways to stop the interruptions of thoughts.*

One way to stop interruptions is to not get

involved with the thoughts or feelings that are nudging you for your attention. Simply acknowledge the interrupting thought, look at it objectively, say to yourself, "*Ahah—there's a thought,*" and let it go. Don't follow it; just look at it. For example, if you think about going to the movies, that's okay. Just acknowledge the fact that you had a thought about going to the movies. But if you follow the thought, you will start to think about when the movie starts, how much time to leave to get there on time, who will go with you, and so on. So don't follow the thought. *Just look at it, and it will go away.*

A second way to deal with an interrupting thought is to begin immediately to concentrate more on the Golden Light. (You will soon learn about this light when you listen to the meditation tape.) Make the Golden Light deeper, warmer and more radiantly pure, and your thoughts will be absorbed into it.

A third effective method to eliminate an intrusive thought is to change it to another. If you divert a thought to a spiritual thought, you will soon be back to the "thoughtless," meditative state. For example, if you begin to think about some project you have to do, change the thought to something like, "God loves me," and say this over and over again. "*God loves me, God loves me, God loves me, God loves me. . .*" Soon you will be back into the meditation.

During the first part of the meditation, be aware that your mind is accustomed to thinking, not to quiet. So even after your mind seems to quiet down, thoughts will pop up frequently. Do not be concerned about this. The three methods described above are all effective to stop the thoughts as they occur. Also, as you begin taking better care of yourself, particularly with better nourishment and regular exercise, the thoughts will automatically become much less likely to occur.

Have a pen or pencil and a piece of paper nearby. Sit comfortably in a chair, on a couch, a bed or on the floor, the grass, the beach, wherever you won't be disturbed. If you hear any sound – a bird, a car horn, children's voices – recognize the sound as just part of your normal environment, and don't dwell on it. Now place your hands gently in your lap and begin to relax. . .

The following is a written description of the taped meditation. If you do not have a tape player then ask someone to read it to you slowly, calmly and peacefully:

"PRESCRIPTION FOR LIFE MEDITATION"

Close your eyes. Take a slow, deep breath through your mouth, and then very slowly, let it out through your nose.

Take another deep breath through your mouth . . . very long and very deep . . . and then very slowly, let it out through your nose.

Take another slow, deep breath through your mouth . . . and while you slowly let it out through your nose . . . begin to relax the muscles behind your eyes.

Take another deep breath through your mouth, and while you very slowly let it out through your nose, begin to relax the muscles at the base of your tongue.

Take another deep breath through your mouth and as you slowly let it out through your nose, begin to relax the muscles of your neck, your shoulders, your arms, your forearms, your hands, and your fingers . . . right down to your fingertips.

Continue breathing now, deeply and regularly, and begin to relax the muscles of your chest and your abdomen.

Breathe deeply again and relax the muscles of your back.

Continue to breathe deeply. Relax the muscles of your buttocks, your thighs, your calves, and your feet and your toes. Breathe and relax.

Begin now to envision a warm, healing, pure, Golden Light entering into all ten of your toes. Feel this warm, healing, Golden Light filling your feet with its radiance and its warmth and making your feet relax.

Now feel the warm, healing, pure Golden Light very slowly rising in your body. Feel it fill your ankles with warmth and with healing. Feel your ankles relax in the light. Feel the light fill all the tendons and ligaments of your ankles. Feel the light filling the entire space of your ankle joints with healing, relaxing, wonderful warmth.

Now feel the warm, healing Golden Light filling your calf muscles. Feel it entering your knee joints and filling the tendons and ligaments of your knees with warmth. Feel the healing warmth of the light relaxing your knees. Feel the entire space of your knee joints filled with warm, healing Golden Light.

Feel the Golden Light very slowly filling your thighs with warmth and healing. Become aware of how much you store up in your muscles all the sadness and little upsets and disappointments of your every day life. Now feel the power of the healing Golden Light to extinguish all the painful, hurtful memories stored within your muscles. Feel the Golden Light fill your muscles and remove the hurtful memories.

Feel the pure, healing Golden Light filling your hip joints with warmth and relaxation. Feel the beautiful Golden Light filling your private areas, and filling your pelvis and all the organs in it. Feel the Golden Light filling the organs with healing, warm, radiant light.

Feel the healing light spreading to your abdomen. Feel the Golden Light filling your intestines from their beginning to their end with healing warmth. Feel the Golden Light fill your bladder and kidneys and liver and spleen. Feel the warm, healing Golden Light filling your stomach, and the entire inside of your abdomen. Feel the warmth, the pureness and the healing energy of the Golden Light.

Now feel the Golden Light appearing in your back. Imagine it filling each and every one of your vertebrae. Feel the warmth of the Light in the discs between the vertebrae and feel the Golden Light spread to the muscles of your back. Let every muscle fiber in your back slowly fill with pure, warm, healing, Golden Light. Feel the Golden Light remove the pain and spasm from all the muscles in your back.

Experience the Golden Light appearing now in your lungs. Feel it filling each and every air sac with warmth and healing and purity.

Then feel the Golden Light appearing in your heart, filling all four chambers with warmth, love, compassion, and healing. Feel the Golden Light filling the muscles of your heart and beginning to course through the coronary arteries. Feel your coronary arteries filled with warmth, and with healing, and with love and compassion and forgiveness and purity and Light.

Feel the Golden Light spreading to your neck, and filling the tendons and ligaments and muscles with warmth and with healing and with total relaxation. Now feel the Golden Light beginning to fill your shoulders, your arms, your elbows, your forearms, your hands, your palms, your fingers, all the way to your fingertips, all filled with warmth and healing Golden Light.

Feel the Golden Light in your mouth now, filling your lips with warmth and with healing. Filling your gums, your teeth, your tongue and your throat. Feel the warmth filling your entire mouth now. Pure Golden Light.

Feel the Light filling your nose and your sinuses with warmth and with healing. Feel the Light filling your cheeks and your ears. Feel the warmth of the Light filling your eyes. Feel the Light filling your brain so that each and every brain cell is filled with pure, radiant, healing Light.

Now your entire body is filled with Golden Light; feel the Light becoming more intense, more radiant, warmer, and more pure. Feel the light becoming so intense that you merge with the light. Merge with the light now.

VERY SILENTLY, AND FOR AS LONG AS YOU WISH, BECOME THE LIGHT. BECOME THE LIGHT. . . . .
. . . . .
. . . . .
. . . . .
. . . . .
. . . . . (SILENCE). . . . .
. . . . .
. . . . .
. . . . .
. . . . .

At this time, begin to picture yourself in a beautiful country meadow on a wonderful, warm sunny day. See yourself standing in green grass surrounded by hundreds of thousands of beautiful wildflowers. See mountains in the background and hear birds singing.

In front of you, in this lovely meadow, see an artist's easel. On the easel see an empty canvas. Now have paints and brushes in your hands and become a perfectly talented and wonderful artist.

Walk up to the easel and take your paints and brushes and begin to paint a picture of your self as healthy and happy and wholesome.

Paint your eyes and your skin as radiant and glowing; paint your muscles and joints as flexible and healthy; paint your body as youthful and trim; paint your bones as vibrant and strong; paint your nervous system as calm and full of health; paint your immune system as strong and resistant and perfectly well.

Paint your organs without dis-ease; paint your body without addictions or pain. Paint yourself in perfect, wonderful, radiant health. Paint an expression on your face of security and contentment.

*SILENTLY NOW, PAINT YOURSELF
WELL..................................*
....
....
....
............(PAINTING SILENTLY)......
....
....
....
....

*At this time, take your brushes and paints
and paint your signature on the lower right
hand corner of the painting. Paint your
signature very clearly, and then put your
brushes and paints down. Begin to walk away
from the easel. . .*

*Walk through the meadow on this warm
summer day until you come to a woods. Begin
to walk through the woods now. See the bright
sunshine illuminating your path. Feel the pine
needles and the twigs underneath your feet as
you walk further into the woods. As you
continue to walk, come to a clearing in the
woods. Look around and see in front of you a
wonderful country cottage.*

*See this "storybook-like" cottage as
peaceful and serene and almost dreamlike in*

its perfection. Walk up to its front door and find it open. Walk into the cottage. Look around and see yourself in a warm, comfortable, peaceful and almost familiar sitting room. See the sunshine streaming through the windows. Now, while you are looking around and feeling peaceful and secure, sit down on a sofa in the middle of the room. Continue breathing deeply and feel the Golden Light within you.

Become aware this time of another presence entering the room through a door behind your left shoulder. Look carefully now and see that this presence is a wise and wonderful Master of Life. Become aware that this Master of Life contains within his heart and soul all the Wisdom of the entire universe. See that this Master of Life radiates pure Love and Grace and Healing and Forgiveness.

See the Master of Life walk over to the couch and see him sit down beside you and look at your face. Feel total Compassion and Forgiveness flowing from the Master as he gazes into your eyes.

Hear the Master of Life tell you he has come to deliver a personal message to you. Hear the Master tell you that the message he has come to give you is about the responsibility it is now appropriate for you to take for your

*own health and well being. . . . .What is
necessary for you to do in order to be more
healthy and well. . .*

   *NOW LISTEN SILENTLY AS THE
MASTER OF LIFE SPEAKS TO YOU
ABOUT YOUR RESPONSIBILITY . . . .*
. . . .
. . . .
. . . .
. . . .
. . . .*(LISTENING SILENTLY)*. . . . .
. . . .
. . . .
. . . .

*Now it is time for the Master to go. Hear
him tell you that he will be present in this
cottage every day so you may visit with him
and gain inspiration and wisdom. See the
Master arise from the couch and leave the
cottage through the same door that he
entered.*

*See yourself rise from the couch and walk
out of the cottage through the front door. Go
back into the woods on this warm, wonderful,
sunny day. Walk back through the woods on
the pine needle trail until you come to the
beautiful meadow where you started.*

*When you are back in the meadow, walk
up to a very tall, old, stately tree. Put your*

*arms around this tall and stately tree. Rest
your cheek against its bark. Now, as you feel
the bark of the tree against your cheek, begin
to feel extremely refreshed and alert. Take a
slow, deep breath, and very slowly open your
eyes. Come back to your waking consciousness.*

Now, take your paper and pen and write down
any ideas that have come to you about how you
can take responsibility for your own health, and
well-being. If nothing has come to you, that's okay;
it will with time – just like learning to drive or ski or
swim.

The process on the meditation therapy tape is
healing in nature. It induces endorphin release, it
assists you in setting attainable goals, and it is
inspiring, so that your inner self can lovingly and
caringly begin whispering to you. The meditation
brings your mind into an alpha or theta state, and
images set in your mind in that state are reflected to
all of the parts of your body.

This *Wellness* and healing process has been
used with patients from ages four to eighty-six, and
has worked wonderfully. It is simple enough to be
practiced with just the aid of the cassette, as long as
you suspend the need to agree or disagree.

The point is, in order to get well and stay
healthy, you must quiet your mind for thirty
minutes each day. Very simple, but essential. This
is the first step across the bridge to *Wellness*.

The special sound technology on the tape

actually helps to balance the function of the right and left hemispheres of your brain. *It is best, if at all possible, to listen to the tape with headphones.* There are portable "Walkman" type tape players with headphones that sell for as little as ten dollars. There is no need to have a fancy machine and if necessary any working tape player will do.

It is easiest to do this meditation first thing in the morning, (and then the health producing images will be sending your body messages all day), but any time is okay as long as you do it *every* day!

Meditation is like prayer, but in prayer we are usually *asking* for something, whereas in meditation we're *listening* for God's answer.

INGREDIENT TWO: EXERCISE

As you may know from past experience, exercise is usually the most difficult step toward good health. Yet virtually every patient I work with credits exercise as the crucial turning point for *Wellness*. They also say they experienced the most resistance and reluctance to get on with this part of their agreement.

If you experience this common resistance to even beginning the exercise section of the bridge, be aware that your ego or "*Thinker*" is now really becoming very threatened by its potential extinction.

The immediate and gratifying results you get from exercise are trouble for your ego. Remember that your ego is merely the sum total of all your beliefs, attitudes, convictions, viewpoints, memories and thoughts. It wants nothing more than to be left alone and undisturbed.

Now, if you are sick and tired, ill not well, down not up, sad not glad, then "I Lack Love" has become a dominant theme in your ego, and your ego will defend itself in any manner it can. People even jump off bridges or hurl themselves out of windows rather than face their egos and deal with the changes that their egos don't want them to make.

No wonder that many, if not most, individuals not already into exercise experience resistance. They begin to *think* that it is okay to skip their exercise today and then tomorrow. It's as if the ego were screaming, "STOP!" because it knows what happens with exercise. "I Lack Love" gives way to "I Love Life."

Why is this? Patients describe exercise as a way to keep their minds clear. They commonly tell me it lets them detach themselves from their thoughts. It enables them to get hold of, to harness, literally to corral the thoughts that disturb them the most.

One of my patients, Jeff Santangelo, was a sixty-year old worried executive with a twenty-year old ulcer that bled every four or five years: After crossing the bridge he stopped his Tagamet and Valium routines. He told me that during the first part of his exercise time he says, *"I don't care to think about the disturbing phone calls any longer.*

I choose to think about wind surfing."

Another patient, forty-year old Anna Hill, was a severe hypochrondriac who was prey to virtually any real or imagined disease – colitis, arthritis, psoriasis and allergy to name only a few. She decided to cross the bridge and was absolutely beside herself with joy when during a flu epidemic she remained the only one in her household to stay well. She told me her exercise enabled her to *control the flow of ideas* that continuously crossed her mind. Her mind was no longer in "overdrive." She said that during her morning jog, she clearly *saw the thought* of becoming ill with the flu begin to cross her mind and she *stopped the thought* "dead in its tracks" with a counter-thought of such immense power it almost seemed like a vision or spiritual experience. She simply *thought*, "I'm *not* going to get sick, and *that's that!"*

When you exercise, you get to the point where just like waking up from a dream, you understand it as a dream and take control of it instead of allowing it to control you. You are given strength because exercise causes your endorphins to flow as your mind clears and your thoughts settle down. This is the effect mentioned earlier, which is often associated with the "runner's high." You don't have to be a triathlon candidate for it to work for you. With a simple choice of some form of exercise that is easily accessible to you – *so that you will do it* – your natural energies become realigned, and you are back in healthful balance, or harmony, on the mental, physical and emotional levels.

No wonder your ego struggles against your agreeing to exercise, and creates sneaky alibis and excuses to thwart your best intentions. It wants to survive as it is, when health is not familiar to it.

One of my patients, Elaine Cohen, 55, perfectly grasped the essence of the problem and dealt with it. She told me exercise was the turning point in overcoming a number of health problems, "even though I resisted exercising for the first five days of my own agreement with myself because I couldn't get to the gym in the snow." (Notice she doesn't say, "I couldn't exercise;" she says, "I resisted." Elaine knows what her ego is up to, consciously or otherwise.) But, she went on, "I finally turned on the television and had a wonderful time exercising with the lady on Channel 4."

If you are not already exercising, it is necessary to tune out your "*Thinker*." Just agree to exercise for the five weeks of the bridge. In no time at all you will look forward to exercising as often and as much as you can.

Exercise is a way to keep the mind clear, and keeping the mind clear is the key to *Wellness*. When the mind is clear, endorphins flow to heal the unhealthful parts of your body including anxious and insecure areas of your brain that *think the thoughts that persistently attack you during your waking and sleeping hours.*

When you are in a state of less than vibrant *Wellness*, the major issue you are dealing with is a lack of love for your body. A major benefit of exercise is heightened respect for your body. You get immediate and definite feedback. You notice results. You feel better. Life is easier. All of a sudden, you can look back and say, "Whew! I was really in trouble. . . I was really out of shape."

Exercise breaks negative patterns, including depression, not laughing, being stressed out, losing hope, worrying. It gives you another window through which to look at yourself. A lot of people have no idea that there is anything better for them. They are in a habit of being unhappy, overweight, insecure, stressed out, and that is just a way of life for them. It goes on for so many years that they don't realize what they can achieve, and how easily. Exercise is the quickest way to get a glimmer of what's out there.

Exercise lowers blood pressure, reduces cholesterol, helps varicose veins, lessens headaches, backaches, constipation, premenstrual symptoms, anxiety and depression. Exercise decreases your fatty deposits and cellulite. It helps relieve your pain, enhances your sex life, brightens your outlook and in almost all instances just makes you feel good. *Why would anyone not exercise? In almost all instances (other than paralysis), the answer is always the same— I Lack Love.*

Exercise, because it gives quick and obvious results, helps insure the success of the Prescription For Life. Unless you see and feel results, you are not going to be enthusiastic about sticking to the program to break your old habits. Exercise provides fast, positive feedback.

Meaningful and effective exercise is really up to

you to define. A lot of people do it using their pulse
to determine how much they are actually working.
You can do that, but don't let the technical or
measuring techniques you've heard or read about
get in your way. Don't give your ego an excuse to
put off exercising. Pick any form of exercise and do
it! Make it enjoyable, work up a sweat and do it until
you are a little out of breath. Do it for at least fifteen
or twenty minutes a day, three, four, five, or six
days a week. Outdoors is great, but indoors is fine.
Whenever you find a reason not to exercise on any
given day, ask yourself what alternatives exist, and
exercise despite your ego's reluctance! Don't *think*
you don't have to do it.

I recommend walking as a terrific exercise for
anyone whose ego likes to resist exercise. Everyone
knows how to walk! It is so natural, so simple, and
so beneficial, you will wonder why you haven't been
enjoying it all these years.

To learn the kind of walking that is the best
exercise, go to a swimming pool! When children
who are running are told to walk, watch what they
do. They walk alright, but they walk quickly,
pumping their arms. No one had to teach them how
to walk quickly, and *you* already know how, too.
When you were a child you exercised naturally and
had to be slowed down! Now you are simply going
to move again!

The process is so simple! Walk quickly with a
jaunty, lengthy, carefree, rhythmic stride. Pick up
your legs and pump your arms. In good weather you
can walk in beautiful surroundings – parks,

beaches, pretty neighborhoods. In bad weather you can walk in shopping malls, in your house, or even outdoors. A lot of people report that they look forward to rain or snow, as their walks bring them closer to nature, bringing them outdoors when they would have otherwise avoided going outside.

If you are not exercising already, start with a brisk fifteen or twenty minute walk at least three or four days of the week. It is best to start slowly, gradually stretching and warming up for a few minutes. Also stop in a gradual manner by slowing down over a few minutes rather than abruptly. Exercise is one part of the five-week journey across the bridge to *Wellness* that will benefit you dramatically and immediately.

Besides your walks, try to get as much movement into your life as you comfortably can while following the Prescription For Life. When you park your car in a lot, park a few rows farther away than you normally would and walk the few extra yards. If you have a choice between walking or driving to run an errand, try to walk more often. In any way you can *think* of, simply try to move your body more throughout the day. Even going to the television instead of using the remote control will help. Whenever you can move your body more, you will reap the rewards of exercise! And when you become accustomed to regular exercise by following the Prescription For Life, you will *want* to move more. You'll stop *thinking* it's boring or you don't have time.

INGREDIENT THREE: ENERGY NUTRITION

Your *"Thinker"* will fight to keep the status quo in your diet much the way it does in regard to exercise. That is why so many people suffer on diets and go through all sorts of martyrdom only to regain the weight they have lost.

A sensible nutrition plan is crucial to being well. For most people, the guidelines recommended by the National Institutes of Health are a good starting point: Cut down on fats, especially saturated fats; eat more whole carbohydrates (fruits, vegetables, whole grain products); eliminate or severely limit alcohol, caffeine, refined sugar, and salt.

Beyond that, I recommend that you follow an eating plan that is simple, offers variety, aids digestion and is delicious. Harvey and Marilyn Diamond's FIT FOR LIFE and Lisa Tracy's THE GRADUAL VEGETARIAN are outstanding nutritional plans that offer all those advantages. Although some of these books' principles fly in the face of orthodox medicine,[3] they have helped millions of people and hurt none.

---

[3] When I went to medical school, really practical nutrition was not included in the curriculum. This was standard until very recently. The study of energy nutrition is still in its infancy as far as traditional Western Medicine is concerned. Traditional Medicine has taught disease repair. We are just now beginning to look at health in terms of body energy that can be helped by live energy from appropriate food and hindered by foreign energy from inappropriate foods.

The idea of eating only fresh fruit or drinking fresh juice before noon, is a smart one. It allows the body a light way to start the day, while providing essential vitamins, minerals, energy and water in a pure form. I've seen tens of thousands of people of all ages become more healthy, energetic and happy when they have given up heavy breakfasts and eaten just fruit in the morning. This is also a safe, effective way to lose weight. During the Prescription For Life, try to eat only fruit in the morning — all types and as much as you want, as long as it's fresh.

It's also a good idea to not *mix* fruit with any other type of food – so don't eat anything else for at least an hour before or an hour after you eat fruit. This includes waiting an hour after dinner for your fruit dessert.

Another essential feature of a *Wellness* eating style is the reduction or elimination of dairy foods. They are high in saturated fats and frequently lead to congestion in the respiratory system. Some people may be concerned about not getting enough calcium if they cut back on dairy. It is important for you to realize that fresh fruits, vegetables, nuts and seeds have abundant calcium, and more importantly, your body can more efficiently store and *use* their calcium. The calcium in dairy products is hard to utilize in your body. Also, sugar foods deplete your calcium reserves no matter how much dairy you eat, and the high phosphorus content of red meat may inhibit calcium absorption. By eating less red meats and by cutting down on sugar, you will get a lot more and be able to use a lot more calcium in your diet than by eating dairy.

Milk is cow secretion. It is for baby calves; it is *foreign energy*. When our bodies are young we have *extra* enzymes and digestive agents to process this foreign energy. When we get past adolescence we *lose* these extra enzymes and milk then causes imbalance in our energy system – dis-ease: congestion, colds, bronchitis, asthma, ear infections, colitis, rashes, diarrhea, constipation, lethargy, and probably a whole list of other dis-eases including atherosclerosis hypertension, coronary artery disease, strokes, arthritis and perhaps even cancer.

"Osteoporosis" has become the new rallying cry of the dairy industry; you can avoid it – but not with milk. A balanced lifestyle with exercise, abundant green vegetables, nuts and seeds (particularly sesame) and the Prescription For Life is the best preventive medicine for osteoporosis. *This isn't what you've been taught to think, but just remember that what you have been taught to think has made us the most overweight, atherosclerotic, hypertensive, gouty, arthritic, headachy, hemorrhoidal, coronary-prone, cancer-ridden, stressed-out population in the history of the world!*

Cut down on oily and fatty foods. The typical American ingests 260 quarts of oil a year. If you put that in your car that weighs dozens of times more than you, it would *slop* over on to the motor, the fan belts, the radiator, the transmission, etc. In your body it also *slops* over into your coronary and brain vessels, your joints and your heart!

Design your meals so that you avoid mixing

flesh with starch at the same meal. This means giving up the old notion of eating rice with fish or a potato with chicken. Eat only the rice or only the fish, only the potato or only the chicken at any one meal. However, whether you chose to eat flesh or starch at that meal, be sure to have it with a salad and with at least one vegetable. You can more easily digest your meals eating this way, and you will feel lighter, though still satisfied.

At first you may *think* that eating this way limits your choices, but you will soon realize that there is hardly any food you have to give up! You will simply eat the rolls and potatoes or the rice and pasta with salad and vegetables. The flesh that used to be *on* a sandwich can be eaten at another meal with salad and vegetables. Once you are familiar with this simple principle, you will find that you can even eat out, as often as you like, and still eat according to these simple rules.

WONDERFUL FLESH ALTERNATIVES

Red meat, besides being full of fat, hormones and antibiotics, takes your body about three days to digest and eliminate. Therefore do not eat red meat more often than every three days. Chicken and fish, especially if fresh, are better for you than red meat and tend to have more energy. (But most chickens are not allowed to even walk around to gain healthful energy before they die, and more than fifty percent may be infected with salmonella bacteria. As for fish, well you know what happens to it if left out for a day at 98.6 degrees temperature and that is what may also happen when fish is in you!)

If you are used to eating flesh every day, you are in for a treat! As you begin to cut down on your flesh meat, you will discover the delicious, satisfying and healthful benefits of potatoes, pasta and rice.[4]

When you start to build meals around potatoes and rice as a main course, you will find that you digest your meals more easily, you feel lighter and less tired after a big meal, you have more energy during the day, and you sleep better at night.

There is something wonderful about the energy in complex carbohydrates like potatoes, pasta and rice. Famines wipe out populations when the potato, wheat and rice crops fail. Whole populations thrive when these crops are abundant.

---

[4]There are a number of excellent cookbooks available that will teach you creative, delicious, nutritious recipes for meals with less flesh. Among the best are THE MOOSEWOOD COOKBOOK and THE ENCHANTED BROCCOLI FOREST by Molly Katzen (Ten Speed Press, Berkeley, CA); THE NEW LAUREL'S KITCHEN by Laurel Robertson, Carol Flinders, and Brian Ruppenthal (Ten Speed Press, Berkeley, CA). A NEW WAY OF EATING by Marilyn Diamond (Warner Books, New York, NY) and HEALTHY FOR LIFE by Edward & Anneli Taub (American Wellness Association, Sausalito, CA).

Forget what traditional "diets" have always warned about the fattening potato! Eat lots of boiled, mashed and baked potatoes (with salads and vegetables) and watch your weight, your energy and your health improve.

Another wonderful alternative to flesh is pasta. Today there are dozens of pastas to choose from, including those made with whole wheat, spinach or tomato, which color them green or red or brown. Pasta is even made with artichoke. With the variety of shapes, textures, and types of pasta available, you can eat any number of filling, delicious pasta-based meals at home or in restaurants. The only thing to watch out for is that old meatball and spaghetti combination. If you can't do without the meatballs then have either meatballs *or* spaghetti at any given meal—just not the same meal. Have either one with a salad and at least one vegetable. Just do not combine flesh with the starch at the same meal. Pasta primavera replaces linguini with clam sauce.

LIVE FOODS

By eating only fruit in the morning and by including salad and vegetables with lunch and dinner, you are increasing your intake of live foods. Just as your life energy is made up of vibrations unique to you, so live foods have their own, natural energy patterns. When you eat foods in their natural, original states, their life energy and yours are completely compatible. When you eat raw nuts, your body can efficiently store and utilize their calcium and other nutrients. When you eat fresh salad greens and sprouts, your body can more easily absorb their vitamins and minerals. When you eat fresh fruit, their abundant life energy imparts life energy to you.

This may be hard to believe, but it's true. If you eat live foods, unaltered by processing (not canned, not refined, not frozen, not irradiated, not processed, not laced with chemical preservatives, not over-cooked) *you can eat until you are no longer hungry and you will not gain weight. You will actually lose weight.* The energy allows your body to burn excess fat.

The closer a food is to its natural state, the better it is for you, the more compatible its life energy is with yours. Cooking, canning, chemicals, irradiation, and even freezing, alters the molecular structure of food. The energy of that food is altered when the food is processed in any of these ways, and your body's energy does not assimilate the new molecular structure, or the new energy pattern as easily. Nature doesn't condense and dehydrate its orange juice or soak its fruits in syrupy sugar and place it in cans.

If you think of live foods as foods whose energy is compatible with your own, and you eat more and more of these live foods, your health will improve dramatically, and your weight will take care of itself. Forget counting calories, and give up the notion of having to eat less. *You can eat abundant quantities of live foods without worrying about your weight!*

Don't mix starches with flesh and include salads and vegetables at every meal. Eat only fruit before noon during the Prescritption For Life. As you go further across the bridge to *Wellness* you will begin to prefer eating this way. Be aware that your ego will resist these changes at first, but like exercise, eating this way will bring fast results. Bend the rules occasionally if you must, but return to eating either starch *or* flesh with salad and vegetables again at the very next meal.

A caveat for pregnant women: Do not embark on this or any other radical change in your diet during pregnancy. Consult your obstetrician for guidelines on your nutrient needs.

Give yourself credit for whatever you're doing right! And don't feel guilty if you backslide a little. You don't have to be a fanatic. A wonderful tenet of Integrative Medicine is: *Do everything in moderation — including moderation!* Remember that we have all been programmed by well-meaning parents, teachers, doctors and nutritionists to believe a lot of things that just aren't so. Many of us have been treated as "Tube Syndrome" children and have grown up that way. Be aware as you progress through your five weeks of the Prescription For Life that your *"Thinker"* is at work. If you find yourself rationalizing about following these simple dietary rules, be alert! Your *"Thinker"* is engaging in sabotage. Eating only fruit in the morning will help you stay on track for the rest of the day.

You have begun enbalming yourself since you began to eat dead food, not live. Its starts with canned baby formula we *"think"* is as full of vitality as what is in the breast. We have become slaves to our tastebuds and our minds have been programmed to take our food and boil it, refine it, process it, microwave it, radiate it, chemicalize it, and *kill it(!)* before we eat it.

These are the nutritional rules to remember for your Prescription For Life.

1. Try eating only fruit until noon. Avoid mixing fruit with other foods. *Wait* one hour before or after eating fruit to eat other food.
2. Have *either* a starch *or* a flesh food at lunch and at dinner, but don't eat starch and flesh at the same meal.
3. Eat vegetables and salad—as much as you want—at lunch and at dinner.
4. Eliminate dairy products, red meat, sugar, salt, alcohol and caffeine as much as you can.
5. Remember that there are no flowing fields of white bread in nature, potato chips do not grow in the ground and pepsi and coke don't flow in the rivers.
6. LIVE AND VITAL FOOD is for LIVE AND VITAL PEOPLE. Avoid frozen, canned, processed, dehydrated, microwaved, preserved, smoked, dried, pulverized, irradiated, *killed* food.

INGREDIENT FOUR: EXTINGUISHING ADDICTION

You are being *abused* by alcohol, tobacco, cocaine, marijuana or other drugs if you need any of them to feel good, if they cause problems at work, in your family or other relationships, or if they bother your conscience or interfere with your physical vitality and fitness.

Even if none of this is true for you, if you are having more than one or two glasses of wine a day, or more than one or two beers, or more than one or two cocktails, or more than two cigarettes, you should cut down.

If you are a substance abuser and want to make the choice to be well, you must commit yourself to stopping and keep the agreement. The most excellent help possible is available for alcoholics through Alcoholics Anonymous and other fine organizations. Start to cure yourself by first recognizing that the addicted mind is the mind you now have to use to stop the addiction – an example of the difficulty of getting from here to there.

But you have no alternate route. It's the only mind you have. So make your choice and try to keep your ego and habits out of it by making the commitment for just five weeks. You will sign your Prescription For Life agreement at the end of Chapter Eight that will embody this commitment. The five weeks are the time needed to rebalance your body as a whole and *reprogram your thoughts*, which are the crucial first steps toward extinguishing your addiction and then readdicting yourself to feeling so good that you can't stop wanting to feel even better. For alcohol and drug abusers, the other sections of the five-week strategy reinforce quitting your addiction. For people who have broken one addiction, alcohol, only to find themselves relying on other addictions, caffeine or tobacco, this voyage to Wellness can be your liberation from these other addictions.

There is nothing more physically harmful than smoking. *You can stop smoking. You can even stop smoking and lose weight at the same time when you follow your health-care agreement and walk across this bridge to Wellness.*

If you smoke and want to stop, the only additional things you must do while following the Prescription For Life, are to cut out *all* red meat from your diet, cut way down on chicken and fish, and get as much sunshine as you can. (Don't get burned.) Beyond these changes, simply agree to follow the *Wellness* contract and meditate and exercise daily, love someone unconditionally, increase your live food intake by eating only fruit before noon and salads and vegetables with either a starch or flesh at meals, and take precautions for safety.

You can make it easier to stop smoking by avoiding smoke-filled rooms and friends who smoke. Spend time in places where smoking is prohibited: go to movies, museums, gyms or health clubs. Breathe fresh air! Smog is like smoke in that it affects every cell of your body and changes your energy so significantly that it is virtually impossible to reach optimum *Wellness* in a smoggy or smokey environment. Visit the woods, beaches, parks and open spaces in your area where there is little traffic and lots of fresh air. Treat yourself well! (And stop *thinking* you have to gain weight.)

Drug abuse and addiction are perfect examples of how disease begins in the mind as a result of our thoughts. For example, people with small to large quantities of cocaine will finish *whatever* quantity they have just as soon and as quickly as they can because when they are "high," their thoughts take on a new and stronger power of their own and the "*Thinker*" merely *thinks* that it would be great to have more and more cocaine, *now*. The person using cocaine merely keeps using more. If the person has a concern about an overdose, then the "*Thinker*" just *thinks* "no, it will be ok."

The alcoholic or even the occasionally inebriated person is also under the control of the "*Thinker*" He or she *thinks* that one more drink would be fine – and that of course is why most alcoholics or drug users "hit bottom" before seeking help.

Marijuana is particularly obnoxious as it propels the "*Thinker*" into new realms of power because of the euphoria it produces and the "*Thinker*" thinking how pleasant and creative everything is. Millions of people, including attorneys, physicians and other professionals who should "know better," are deluded by their *thoughts* into smoking marijuana two or three times a week – they are *always* under the influence of the drug since it takes three or four days to leave their system.

Whenever the marijuana starts to leave the body, the *"Thinker"* thinks that it's time to smoke again—"after all it's been three or four days so what harm could there be?"

The *"Thinker"* of the drug abuser or alcoholic develops a power of its own. This is the main problem in the use of even "recreational" amounts of alcohol and drugs. If the user is stressed and the drug is enjoyable, then the *"Thinker"* is unleashed on a wild ride that may become a lifelong spree.

If you are an alcoholic or if you are using cocaine, marijuana, uppers, downers or any other "recreational" drug, most likely you began because it made you feel good. Now you require it in order not to feel sick. If you can't stop or won't stop it is time to take yourself to one of the self-help organizations designed to help you out of the fix you are in. Seek professional help.

Recognize that if you had not needed the substance to feel good, you would not have used it in the first place. A friend of mine, a former addict, has a wonderful phrase: *"Your inner works need fixing."* The prime avenue of release for you is through self-responsibility, self-value, self-esteem and a higher regard and reverence for life.

Your life energy has been chemically dependent on a foreign energy for too long! Get your endorphins flowing and discover how your own life energy can keep you feeling good all the time.

INGREDIENT FIVE: SELF-SAFETY

This section of the bridge is the easiest to cross, yet many people will be surprised at how their egos will try to circumvent even this simple and basically common-sense agreement. *Buckle your seat belt and make sure your passengers do likewise before you pull away from the curb.* Obey traffic laws, including speed limits.

To cross through the safety section on the bridge to *Wellness* you must become aware of potential dangers in your environment and what you can do to minimize them.

If you have a young child, your pediatrician may have given you a list of household hazards and ways to eliminate them. These include: moving all cleaning chemicals and other dangerous substances up high and out of reach; safely blocking access to steps and similar dangers; blocking unused electrical outlets; removing poisonous plants; keeping appliances and sharp tools out of reach; being alert for heavy objects that could fall or tip over and for dangerous things a child could climb on.

Whether or not you have a child living with you, a few simple measures will make your life safer. Remove obvious fire hazards and have a working smoke alarm, a fire extinguisher and a rehearsed emergency fire escape route. Also assess your work place for dangers and pollutants. There may be conditions outlawed by OSHA, in which case you may have to crusade for change or consider changing jobs. (*Ms.* Magazine in 1986 reported that hazardous chemicals in California's Silicon Valley were causing problems ranging from depression to life-threatening conditions. Many women left those jobs, but perhaps too late.)

Other occupational hazards can be eliminated more simply. Marianne, a newspaper reporter, was a nonsmoker surrounded by smokers. She and the other nonsmokers in the office were constantly complaining that they couldn't breathe. Marianne nagged the building services department with a series of phone calls and memos until finally someone came to examine the ventilation system. They discovered the exhaust vents under the radiators were clogged with about an inch of tobacco-colored dust! After a half-hour cleaning, the vents did their job and the nonsmokers could breathe a little easier.

Whatever it takes, arrange your life so that you are taking fewer risks with it.[5] Begin by wearing seat belts and driving safely. If you find yourself resisting seat belts, remember that this is your ego at work. Seven out of ten deaths from automobile accidents can be avoided with seat belts. If you won't take three seconds to buckle up –at least for the next five weeks — you are lacking love for yourself. You must overcome the "*Thinker*." The other steps across the bridge will help you.

---

[5] Practical Guide To Survival, by Victoria Mason, (Mason/Slawson, 1987), is an excellent guide to preventing and dealing with disasters in the home.

INGREDIENT SIX: LOVINGNESS

The Prescription For Life requires that you show unconditional love to someone in your life. Begin to think of what personal relationship you can enhance. With whom can you start a new and better relationship? With which person could you be more positive, open, disclosing, caring and loving? A husband, wife, child, parent, grandparent, grandchild or other relative? A friend, teacher, rabbi, priest, minister, doctor, boss, employee or co-worker, store-keeper, neighbor? Anyone you can think of with whom you could be more caring and to whom you could show unconditional kindness and love.

In the event that there is no one in your life, no person even to reach by long distance phone or by letter, then buy, borrow or adopt a puppy or kitten. This will assure that there will be no possible obstacle to this very important step on the bridge to Wellness.

Unconditional love simply means to respect and love the other person as they are, no matter what they do or say or how they behave or in what manner they respond or relate to you. It means you do not judge them, become upset or angry with them, get disappointed by their reaction to you, or attempt to change who they are or what they act like. Don't set up expectations about how they will or won't behave; you don't even have to wonder why they do the things they do. Just accept them.

You're not being asked to love or even like the person's beliefs or behavior or choices or attitudes – only to move beyond evaluating and criticizing and judging, and to love the person for who he or she is.

Unconditional love is a special attitude that clearly conveys kindness, caring and respect. You will have your own ways of demonstrating that you care. It is only necessary that you keep it unconditional — without strings attached – and that it last for the span of the bridge you are crossing (five weeks).

Part of this step involves actively demonstrating your love in some way. You can do this in words – uttered in person, by phone, or by letter. You can imply your feeling with a smile or a gift or a gesture or a letter or a phone call, or some type of assistance *as long as it is clear that something special is occurring.* You will know if it is clear, and you will know if you are unnecessarily withholding your efforts because of a lack of unconditional love on your part. You will know if you are living up to this part of the agreement. Your efforts can be large or small – a love letter to a child away from home or a grandparent far away and lonely; a reaffirmation of love to a husband or wife – complimenting, admiring, respecting, and even more important, accepting in total the person you know he or she really is, the one you loved in the very first place.

It is the *gist* of this agreement that is important. You must not judge, evaluate or try to change the person's behavior, or act or communicate in any way that is not kind, helpful, accepting and loving.

You don't have to be sickly sweet or fawning or even particularly obvious to fulfill this part of the Prescription For Life. You will know in your heart if you are doing it.

An important result of your unconditional love will be that you will have to open your heart completely to the other person and accept the care, praise, or love he or she may unconsciously or consciously radiate *back to you.* You must accept the results of your efforts, and accept whatever love may be returned. Sometimes the love that is returned may be embarrassingly plentiful, or it may be scant and difficult to detect. The unconditionality of your love will neutralize your embarrassment or your disappointment. Just keep your heart open and accept whatever comes your way. *Be receptive* and know that you are living up to your agreement.

This ingredient can be especially effective if you chose to unconditionally love a person you are in conflict with. Cready Erwin a philosopher and teacher, notes that although we blame our conflicts on other people, no one can make us feel or think the way we do. *We alone are responsible for our feelings. We respond to people and to situations on the basis of our own ego, experiences, thoughts, and attitudes—in other words, our "Thinker."*

If, when anger occurs, we take a step back from the situation, we begin to see that the other person may just have the very traits we dislike in ourselves. Often, you will find that you and the other person are really complimentary to each other—not mortal enemies.

Love, faith, laughter and hope are consistently the greatest healing factors I see in my clinical work. As a scientist, I have sometimes felt almost bypassed by all of it, yet cannot deny its prevalence and power.

This ingredient of the Prescription For Life will be easier to follow than your "*Thinker*" may think because of the personal value and self-esteem you are going to develop with the Prescription For Life. You are, by nature, driven to connect with others in loving, sharing ways. Developing personal esteem helps you feel *entitled* to be surrounded by friendly and supportive people and your confidence will enable you to receive love and have your love accepted in return.

By loving someone in your life with unconditional love, by forgiving anyone who is meaningful in your life –extinguishing the anger buried in your body and releasing its energy for more useful purposes – and by opening your heart unconditionally to receive love back, you begin loving yourself, you begin to replace the old programming of "I Lack Love" with "I Love Life."

INGREDIENT SEVEN: ETHICAL LIVING

As you progress on the bridge to *Wellness*, you will notice how most of your behavior is *self-reinforcing*. As you eat according to the simple principles of fruit in the morning, not eating flesh with starch and more live food consumption, you will find that you *want* to eat that way more and more. As you meditate every day, you will find that you *want* to meditate every day. As you exercise, you will *want* to exercise. Behavior that makes you feel good is self-reinforcing.

Yet so is behavior that is bad for you! If you skip a day of exercise, it becomes easier to justify skipping another. If you choose not to meditate one day, your *"Thinker"* will more easily allow you to not meditate the next day by *thinking* it is not convenient or unnecessary.

The same is true for ethical behavior. A major characteristic of *Wellness* is feeling good about yourself. When you are living your life in an ethical way, ethical behavior is self-reinforcing. You feel good about the way you treat yourself and others. You have nothing to hide, and nothing to be ashamed of.

Do nothing wrong for the next five weeks. If you are not sure something may be wrong then don't do it. It is easy to continue living ethically when you take time to appreciate how good you feel by doing what is right. This may involve simply sticking to your health-care agreement, or it may mean telling the cashier when he's made a small error in your favor. Maybe even picking up an empty beer can on the beach that wasn't yours. *(How about not even looking in someone else's medicine chest when you're in their bathroom?)*

Whatever it takes, during the Prescription For Life you must act ethically and feel good about the way you treat yourself and others. "Do unto others as you would have others do unto you," is aptly named the Golden Rule. The confidence, peace and good feelings it effects will adorn you with an inner glow and sense of wellbeing more valuable than gold. It is unfortunate that while we have cracked the secret of the atom we have forgotten the "Ten Commandments" and discarded the "Sermon on the Mount."

For the next five weeks, be committed to the following rule: *Do nothing you know to be wrong, and refrain from doing anything if you are not sure if it may be wrong.* Your self-value will be raised and reinforced, your endorphins will flow and your good health will reflect an inner and outer sense of well-being. *Remember that in this age of stress, health is determined by self value, personal responsibility and reverence for life.*

Meditation, exercise, nutrition, safety, deaddiction, lovingness, and ethical behavior. These are the seven steps across the bridge from sick and tired. Walk on!

Chapter Nine

Your *Wellness* Contract

YOUR *WELLNESS* CONTRACT

E arly in your voyage to *Wellness* you tested your Response-ability Quotient for *Wellness* with the "Response-Ability Scale." It is almost time to take the first step onto the bridge to *Wellness*, to actively engage yourself in the pursuit of signing a well-being health care agreement with yourself.

The physical act of signing the agreement helps you across the bridge. Do not THINK you don't have to sign the agreement. It will very effectively keep you from faltering and just quietly backsliding into defeat.

When you sign your agreement you get to confront not only your ego and your "I Lack Love" programming, but your mortality itself. It is like drawing aside a curtain in your mind so you can see clearly how your choices make you ill or keep you well.

If possible, send or give a copy to your doctor to become part of your medical records. Also, give a copy of the agreement to a loved one or a good friend who is willing to act as an ally—*your personal health facilitator.*

Here's how it works. During your five-week

Prescription For Life you must keep a very simple daily record (See page 243). Writing **YES** or **NO** under the date every day is all you need to do. If you see by your records that you are beginning to falter in your agreement, then you *must* discuss it with your health ally and follow his or her judgement as to whether your faltering is justifiable or not. If you have sprained your ankle, for example, your ally would tell you that obviously you cannot exercise until it is better. If you have overslept and not been able to exercise before work because your alarm clock isn't working, your health ally would tell you that you are being dishonest. *If possible, have your personal health facilitator call you at least twice a week to ask about your progress. Or call him or her yourself to check in.*

The health-care agreement spells out in detail what you are willing to do to become healthy and stay well. You simply write down what you are willing to do in the areas of nutrition, exercise, meditation, safety, lovingness, chemical substance abuse and ethical behavior. Then, on your honor and as a commitment to yourself and your loved ones, you sign it and distribute your copies. Your agreement is all you need as you begin your Prescription For Life.

Remember, *Wellness* is your choice. You can increase control of your health destiny but you may not be ready to do so. Although we all say we would do *anything* to get well it is amazing how our *"Thinker"* thinks—"Oh, but I'm not willing to do *that!* (exercise, eat better, live ethically, meditate, etc). When you *are* ready to choose *Wellness*, then you will sign the agreement knowing and believing that you are ready to cross the bridge.

The health-care agreement is your acceptance of responsibility for who you are and what you want to be. Love yourself, and rejuvenate, regenerate and re-integrate. *At-one-ment*, not atonement.

Now here is a bonus that will overcome any last minute doubts you may have. *It is only necessary for you to comply with eighty percent of your own promises.* If, once in a while you forget to love your person unconditionally, you can forgive yourself; you will not "blow it," as long as you return to your commitment immediately. If once a week or so you do not meditate, or eat properly, you will *not* sabotage your agreement. You will know and your health ally will know if you are really complying with your agreement. In general all your good vows and your ethical behaviour will be self-reinforcing and you will *want* to comply much more than eighty percent!

Make your choice now. If you are willing, make your choice to be healthy into a commitment for life. It begins with day "one" of a short, five-week voyage to *Wellness*.

The *Wellness* contract follows *but you will not sign it until the end of the first week*. Look at it and agree to it, but then continue to read about the last hurdle. To correctly follow your Prescription For Life it is crucial that you listen to the meditation therapy tape for at least five days. *After* you have listened to the tape for five days, then you must sign the Wellness Contract. Do not sign the contract unless you have listened to the meditation therapy tape for 5 days.

Rx
FOR
LIFE

WELLNESS
CONTRACT

I,_____, hereby agree to invest myself in the pursuit of *Wellness* for the next five weeks as described in the following contract:

Article 1. Nutrition:

To eat more life foods; to eat only fruit until noon; to eat salad and vegetables with lunch and dinner; to eat either starch or flesh at lunch and dinner but not both at the same meal; to reduce my intake of red meat, sugar, salt, canned foods, dairy products and coffee — *this is optimal.*

This is what I am willing to do for the next five weeks:

. . . .

. . . .

. . . .

Article 2. Exercise:

To schedule and pursue at least twenty minutes of vigorous exercise five or six days a week. To walk briskly for twenty minutes or substitute a preferred exercise — *this is optimal.*

This is what I am willing to do for the next five weeks.

. . . .

. . . .

. . . .

Article 3. Meditation:

To quiet my mind at approximately the same time every day for at least twenty minutes, and to take notes immediately afterwards on the steps I can take to take charge of my own health destiny:

I *am* willing to do this for the next five weeks:

. . . .

. . . .

Article 4. Safety:

To use seat belts and to drive safely within the speed limit.

I will do this and I am also willing to do the following for the next five weeks:

. . . .

. . . .

Article 5. De-Addiction:

To seek genuine help to end my dependence on drugs, alcohol, tobacco, caffeine, and other chemical substances.

This is what I am willing to do:

. . . .

. . . .

Article 6. Lovingness:

To love someone unconditionally.

This is who I will love unconditionally:

. . . .

Article 7. Ethical Behavior:

To do nothing that is wrong and to avoid doing anything that I suspect may be wrong. To act towards others as I would want them to act toward me.

This I am willing to do for the next five weeks:

. . . .
. . . .

Article 8. (Fill In):

This is what I am also willing to do for the next five weeks:

. . . .
. . . .

I promise on my honor* and integrity, to achieve a level of at least 80% in complying with the specifications of this contract.

Signed: _____ Date: _____

Witnessed: _____ Date: _____
          (Your health ally or your doctor)

Date five weeks from now: _____

*"**On your honor**" **means that you are making an absolute commitment to yourself and to a Higher Power. Your vow is sacred. Signing your name to this document means you** *will* **assume personal responsibility for control of your health destiny.**

A WORD ABOUT GUILT AND BLAME

Practitioners of Integrative Medicine *never* blame sick people for being ill. This is not what the Prescription For Life is about.

Of course there are some people who may not recover in the traditional sense of becoming unsick. They must not feel guilty. What is important to remember about Integrative Medicine is that it addresses *dis-ease*, not just disease. *Everyone* can improve the quality of his or her life. This is the goal of the Prescription For Life.

Remember that *Wellness* means balanced body, mind, and soul. This Prescription For Life *will* enhance the quality of life. You will certainly not be harmed by anything in this Prescription For Life, the aim of which is to establish within you a loving awareness of who you really are. All illnesses can teach us something, and if that lesson is meant to be an acceptance of our mortality, then this Prescription For Life will help us accept that with grace and with ease.

The integration of body, mind, and spirit is what life is all about. Integrative Medicine is a return to a system of medical care that accepts this as natural. Sickness is not right or wrong, good or bad. No guilt is involved. Even though most illness today occurs prematurely due to stress, detrimental habits and environmental hazards, we would be foolish to believe that we can forever challenge our mortality. We are part of Nature's vast scheme to rebuild and replenish itself; just as fields of flowers must wilt so that others can grow. What this Prescription For Life offers you is a chance to understand your part in this vast scheme, and an opportunity to enjoy your role to the fullest. To be fully alive and to live well is the goal here.

Chapter Ten

The Last Hurdle

T here is a final holdout programmed into you. It surfaces when *Wellness* is just within your grasp. Your ego and *"Thinker,"* in a last-ditch effort to defend itself, will slowly reveal a perfectly rational sequence of thoughts to allow you, gradually and gracefully, to bow out of your commitment to yourself.

This is the way the last-ditch survival mechanism works. You have made your commitment to assume the responsibility for *Wellness*. You are inwardly convinced you are on the right path. You have calmly signed your *Wellness* Contract. And you then very nonchalantly begin putting off doing what you have agreed to do.

Gradually and gracefully, you start to falter in one of your promised behaviors. Just one. You then find yourself not taking the steps necessary to fulfill a second . . . and then a third.

Before you know it, feeling perfectly calm and rational about what you are about to do, you dismiss yourself, without guilt or recrimination, from the entire agreement, forget what you have learned, and go on your usual way. Later, you wonder what happened.

What happened is that the ego, your *"Thinker,"* a wonderous mechanism, looked out for itself. When outright resistance to health induction fails and debate won't work and your excuses aren't believable to even you, your ego quietly, gradually and without challenge, removes you from the fray and excuses you from your promises. It lets you out of school, so to speak. It sends you off on a holiday.

It is now extremely important that you begin to extinguish the program in your ego that subverts the choices you made to be healthy. After all, you made those choices because at a deep, inner level you knew they were necessary.

Extinguishing the program that allows your ego to let you off the hook requires only your recognizing that it's there. Your ego's powerful survival mechanism can be neutralized simply by your being aware of its presence and negativism.

To keep your eye on the negative aspects of the ego's behavior, it helps to remember where they come from. The source of the negative programming and conditioning is the *I Lack Love* syndrome, compounded by the "S Factor" and the attitude of *atonement* instead of at-one-ment. Aknowledge this, and then go back to practicing your lovingness, exercise, nutrition, meditation, drug-free lifestyle, safety, and ethical behavior. Remind yourself and your *"Thinker"* that you are on your own honor to live up to your own vows and fulfill your own commitments. Don't say, *"I'm trying"* or *"I think I can"* or *"I should"*—say *"I WILL."*

The philosophers of the new age have what they

call the Gaia theory (Gaia was the Greek Mother Earth goddess) which holds that the environmental outrages perpetrated on one part of the planet effect the entire planet, its atmosphere and ecosystem. In this second half of the twentieth century we have become all too aware, to our sorrow, of our ability to make the Earth sick with poisonous wastes.

We discussed earlier how the smoke you inhale and in a similar fashion, the foods you eat, or the x-rays you absorb are reflected in the health of your every cell, and in every part of your body, even down to your smallest toenail. Just as we are unique forms of energy, so everything on the planet is a unique form of energy. All matter is energy. We are all energy.

Believe it! But don't be immobilized by it. Just as one part of the body communicates dis-ease to the whole, so can one part impart *Wellness* throughout. The effects of good health can be cumulative, even geometric.

I believe in you. I know you can do it. I know you want to do it. I have seen it happen tens of thousands of times — in people who are now bounding with energy. There is not a single one of you who can't make it. Your illness or your *Wellness* is so much a matter of your attitudes and the *thoughts* you think with. Your body and your mind have the power to reverse illness and dis-ease.

You are about to embark on a journey to understand the importance of thought in health and dis-ease. You are going to witness personally the sickness-combatting, life-extending, stress-reducing properties of the healing chemicals in your body. What a wonderful power your mind has to make you well! Walk on!

Chapter Eleven

Week by Week Overview

Week One

Your first week involves just reading this book, quietly contemplating the fact that you have decided to take control of your health destiny and listening to the meditation therapy tape.

Besides reading and thinking about your journey towards *Wellness*, all you have to do this week is meditate. Make sure to jot down any feelings, thoughts, notions and revelations that occur to you after you open your eyes. This requires only twenty minutes a day to listen to the meditation therapy tape and write down your impressions.

Even if you don't feel you have the time or don't *think* you would be interested, or that this will work for you, make a commitment to do it anyway. Any negative thoughts or feelings, any doubts about whether or not this is for you, are simply a reflection of your ego and *"Thinker"* not wanting to change; don't let these thoughts stop you! The meditation therapy tape itself will help reprogram your thoughts so that optimism can replace doubt, and *Wellness* will replace dis-ease.

Finally, every day this week, write a simple "yes" or even just a check next to each day in the following record keeping system, to credit yourself with having begun.

Do not do more than what is prescribed. You cannot push awareness, and you cannot force *Wellness*. Slowly, as your behavior changes, your health will change.

You are embarking on a tremendous adventure.

You are going to be *WELL*. It seems stranger than fiction but it is not. You must take your steps just one at a time.

DO NOT GO ON TO WEEK TWO UNTIL YOU HAVE LISTENED, AS DIRECTED, TO THE MEDITATION THERAPY TAPE FOR AT LEAST FIVE DAYS.

Rx FOR LIFE

DAILY RECORD

Week One

**Please do not go any further until you have
meditated for at least five days.**

	day 1	day 2	day 3	day 4	day 5	day 6	day 7
enter day of the week							
Meditation Listening to tape, Writing notes							

(Just write down "yes" or "no.")

Week Two

Begin week two by filling out and *signing* your *Wellness* agreement. Give a copy to a loved one, a friend, or an acquaintance who will be your health ally. Also, send a copy to your physician to file with your records. *Tell him you are pursuing Wellness!*

Go slowly this week. *Do not do more than what is prescribed.* You absolutely cannot hurry awareness. Simply follow the Prescription For Life, and let awareness come to you.

MEDITATE every day this week, remembering to write down after each meditation what you can do to take better care of yourself.

EXERCISE for at least fifteen minutes for three days this week. If you are already exercising more than that, just keep it up. But do not be overly ambitious. Walking briskly for fifteen minutes three days this week is all you need to do. (Don't forget to warm up and cool down gradually).

NUTRITION this week consists of eating only fresh fruit until noon every day. Eat salad or a vegetable sandwich[6] with lunch, a salad and vegetables with dinner. Avoid mixing any flesh food with pasta, rice, bread, or potato at the same meal.

---

[6] Example: Whole wheat bread with honey mustard (⅓ Dijon mustard, ⅓ honey, ⅓ lemon juice) lettuce, cucumbers, avocado, alfalfa sprouts and sliced tomatoes.

SAFETY precautions begin this week. Wear your seat belt every time you are in a car and insist that passengers buckle up too. Obey the speed limit when you are driving.

ETHICAL BEHAVIOR means you should not do anything you know to be wrong, and do not do anything you suspect might be wrong. Starting this week, pay more attention to the small and large actions in your life, and try to follow this simple rule.

LOVINGNESS begins this week by loving someone in your life unconditionally. Love that person as he or she is without judging.

DE-ADDICTION begins this week as well. If drugs or alcohol are causing a problem at home or where you work, or if you suspect you may have trouble cutting down or quitting, now is the time to seek help. Begin by cutting back 50%, and if this proves impossible amend your *Wellness* agreement to include a commitment to seek professional help with your habit. Do the same for cigarettes. Also for caffeine, ice cream and chocolate.

Week Two

★ **Begin Week Two by filling out and signing your *Wellness* Agreement.**

★ **Change the nutrition commitment to one *you* are more comfortable with, but make it healthful.**

	day 1	day 2	day 3	day 4	day 5	day 6	day 7
enter days of the week							
Meditation Listening to tape, Writing notes							
Nutrition More live food than dead Only fruit before noon Salad and vegetable at lunch and dinner Starch OR flesh							
Exercise Fifteen minutes or more at least three days (Brisk walk or equivalent)							
Safety Seat belts Speed limit							
De-addiction Cutting down 50% or seeking help							
Lovingness Unconditional loving							
Ethical Behavior Doing nothing wrong							

Week Three

Continue MEDITATING every day.

EXERCISE four days this week (unless you are regularly doing more than that).

Continue EATING properly: no flesh foods and starch at the same meal, salads and vegetables at lunch and dinner, fruit until noon.

Pay attention to what you say as well as what you do when you examine your ETHICAL BEHAVIOR.

Continue UNCONDITIONAL LOVING-NESS, SAFETY PRECAUTIONS AND LESS-ENING ADDICTION.

Check in with your personal HEALTH ALLY TO REPORT YOUR PROGRESS.

Week Three

★ **Report your progress to your personal health ally.**

	day 1	day 2	day 3	day 4	day 5	day 6	day 7
enter days of the week							
Meditation Listening to tape, Writing notes							
Nutrition More live food than dead Only fruit before noon Salad and vegetable at lunch and dinner Starch OR flesh							
Exercise Fifteen minutes or more at least four days (Brisk walk or equivalent)							
Safety Seat belts Speed limit							
De-addiction Cutting down 50% or seeking help							
Lovingness Unconditional loving							
Ethical Behavior Doing nothing wrong							

Week Four

As you continue loving someone unconditionally this week, try to appreciate *more* people in your life. Try to accept them for who they are, what they are, as they are, wherever they are in their own lives.

Continue meditating, eating properly, living safely, loving unconditionally and living ethically.

Exercise for *twenty* minutes, *five* times during the week, or as many times as you promised in your health care agreement.

Week Four

★ **Increase your exercise to 5 days this week.**

	day 1	day 2	day 3	day 4	day 5	day 6	day 7
enter days of the week							
Meditation Listening to tape, Writing notes							
Nutrition More live food than dead Only fruit before noon Salad and vegetable at lunch and dinner Starch OR flesh							
Exercise Twenty minutes or more at least five days (Brisk walk or equivalent)							
Safety Seat belts Speed limit							
De-addiction Cutting down 50% or seeking help							
Lovingness Unconditional loving							
Ethical Behavior Doing nothing wrong							

Week Five

You're almost there! This week you will exercise five days again, or as many as you agreed to in your contract. Continue to eat properly and meditate daily (remembering to write down after each session what you can do to take better care of yourself).

Continue loving someone *unconditionally* and accepting as many people in your life as you can, loving them as they are, for who they are.

If you have been seeking help for addiction to drugs, alcohol, tobacco or caffeine, use the meditation and exercise this week to reinforce your commitment to deaddiction.

Safe driving should be habitual by now, but pay special attention to the loving message you give yourself every time you buckle up.

Rx FOR LIFE

Week Five

	day 1	day 2	day 3	day 4	day 5	day 6	day 7
enter days of the week							
Meditation Listening to tape, Writing notes							
Nutrition More live food than dead Only fruit before noon Salad and vegetable at lunch and dinner Starch OR flesh							
Exercise At least twenty minutes for five days (Brisk walk or equivalent)							
Safety Seat belts Speed limit							
De-addiction Cutting down 50% or seeking help							
Lovingness Unconditional loving							
Ethical Behavior Doing nothing wrong							

Conclusion

Welcome to the other side! If your experience following your Prescription For Life was like that of almost every one of my patients, you feel terrific, you look terrific, and your life is running more smoothly than it did before. Welcome to physical fitness, mental peace, emotional calm and spiritual tranquility!

You now know that daily meditation reinforces *health-inducing* thoughts, and you are in the habit of strengthening your inner healing force with daily meditations.

Your exercise habit will soon become a healthy addiction if it hasn't already.

Your unhealthy addictions and substance abuses are no longer interfering with your personal energy.

Your ability to love is at its strongest, and you are giving and receiving abundant love to and from yourself and others.

You are eating mostly live foods and combining them properly for maximum health, ease of digestion and optimum weight control.

Every time you get into a car you are reinforcing your love for yourself, your respect for your life, and your concern for the safety of yourself and others.

Your ethical behavior is a natural part of life that makes you feel good and reinforces the beneficial effects of every other aspect of your life.

New people are attracted to you because of your honesty and integrity and the good feelings you give them. You are attracted to new people because of their honesty and integrity, and the good feelings they give you.

If you were to answer the Response-Ability scale on page 76 again you would see that your life style and your reverence for life are what will keep you healthy for the rest of your life.

Remember, the choice is always yours! If your heart is a lock, then your mind is its key. You can turn the key in either direction: Choose *atonement* or *at-one-ment; I Lack Love* or *I Love Life; dark* or *light; sick* or *well; dis-ease* or *ease; discord* or *harmony.* Your unique, personal attitudes are what make up your *"Thinker"* and you now know the behavior patterns and have the awareness to keep that ego watching out for your best interests. Don't forget how stubborn and tenacious your *"Thinker"* is! It will protect the status quo at all costs! Now that your status quo is a healthy, anabolic daily affirmation of life and health, your ego is your best ally!

I would love to hear from you about your experience with the Prescription For Life. Please write to me at:

The American Wellness Association
3030 Bridgeway
Sausalito, California 94965

I am so happy for you! May you continue to live life fully and enjoy the *Wellness* that is always your option! Walk on!

Epilogue

U.S. Health Care Spending Continues Sharp Rise

By MILT FREUDENHEIM

Despite years of efforts to control costs, spending on health care continues to increase far faster than the inflation rate.

Americans spent $500 billion on health care in 1987, a 9.8 percent increase over 1986, the Department of Health and Human Services announced yesterday. The inflation rate for 1987 was 4.4 percent.

What is more, Federal economists estimate that health care will cost the nation $541 billion this year, up 8.2 percent from 1987. And the total will rise 9.1 percent to $590 billion in 1989.

"Medical costs in this country are out of control," said David F. D'Alessandro, president of the corporate sector of the John Hancock Mutual Life Insurance Company in Boston.

Indeed, health spending accounted for 11.1 percent of the gross national product in 1987, up from 9.1 percent in 1980, and some experts see it rising to 15 percent in the 1990's. That increases in this area of spending are almost twice the general inflation rate, which has been between 4 and 5 percent for two years, is a reflection not only of higher prices but of greater use of medical services.

To be sure, Americans want good health care, said Dr. William L. Roper, the Federal Medicare administrator. But "underneath that, there is widespread doubt among individuals and national leaders," he said. "We're not getting full value. We need to do a better job of spending this large amount of money. How do we get better value — for example, improving our infant mortality record — without devoting more money to health care."

Finding a way to restrain costs will be "a major focus of the new Administration and Congress," Dr. Roper said.

Health-care economists, insurance executives and senior Government offi-

Continued on Page 8, Column 1

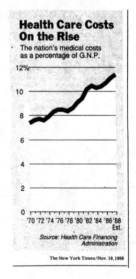

Health Care Costs On the Rise

The nation's medical costs as a percentage of G.N.P.

'70 '72 '74 '76 '78 '80 '82 '84 '86 '88
Est.

Source: Health Care Financing Administration

The New York Times/Nov. 19, 1988

COST AVOIDANCE

Prescription For Life opens an entirely new dimension in health care cost containment — *cost avoidance.* It has always struck me as rather peculiar that the highly intelligent and accomplished individuals running our nation's corporations and labor unions continue to accept the unnecessary and outrageous situation that costs their organizations between three and five hundred dollars a month *per employee.* General Motors recently spent more for health care costs than for steel in the cars they manufacture.

A spate of new solutions arose during the 1980's—prepaid and discounted fee for service plans called PPO's, HMO's and IPA's. Each of these types of organizations have managed to provide only a temporary stop gap to rapidly rising health care costs. Most of the time the dollars saved were just redistributed back to the HMO, PPO, or IPA. Now that big business owns so many hospitals and doctors offices, a poor situation has occurred: stock prices and company earnings go up only as more people get sick—*not a good scheme to lower health care costs!*

Our medical system does not deliver health but it is an excellent disease repair system. The only way to effectively contain health care costs is to keep people well in the first place — *cost avoidance.!*

LETS PUT ILLNESS INTO PERSPECTIVE:

Approximately eighty percent of illnesses are *not* helped with medication, radiation, or surgery. The Surgeon General of the United States declared that the health of the American people will be determined by what they are willing to do for themselves rather than what others do *for* them.

If you are ill you have approximately a ten percent chance of being helped by drugs, radiation or surgery. You *also* have about a ten percent chance that your illness is the *result* of treatment you have received—side affects of drugs and radiation and mishaps of surgery.

Your illness is almost always due to *some* type of stress or detrimental life style that lowers your resistance to disease. Stress is *not* what is happening to you (your job, your spouse, your kids, etc). Stress results from your reaction or response to what is happening. Stress is almost always related to your attitude, lifestyle and habits.

In order to receive the best chance of cure it is necessary to have faith and trust in a physician who not only commands an intimate knowledge of disease but who also has excellent communication skills and is willing to work with you as a partner to control your health destiny. It is necessary for *you* to become actively responsible for enhancing your own healing forces.

Stress is the *real* killer "virus" of our age as it overcomes and defeats the homeostatic forces that keep disease templates dormant. *A key factor therefore in the treatment of dis-ease is the reversal of stress.*

Stress can be reversed through one of three paths: (1) faith in a Higher Power, (2) understanding energy, or (3) accepting the precepts of Psychoneuroimmunology:

Faith in a Higher Power will lead to God taking one hundred steps toward you for every step you take towards Him; for every tear you cry He wipes away a thousand. You can become totally, absolutely and permanently, forgiven. Seeking *Wellness* through the path of faith requires you to begin each day with love, fill each day with love and end each day with love. Your signed Wellness Contract gets you started.

Understanding Energy will lead you to the inevitable conclusion that all you *are* is energy. You are what you think, what you see, what you hear, what you eat and what you breathe. You are a reflection of everything in your environment-everything and everyone around you. *Wellness* through understanding energy comes about through your choices to keep your energy balanced—by meditation, proper nutrition, reduction of drugs and chemicals, exercise, clean air and sensible exposure to the sun's healing rays. Your signed Wellness Contract is your beginning.

Accepting Psychoneuroimmunology will make you aware that your mind ultimately controls your immune system. You feel the way you think. How you feel and think can suppress or enhance your resistance and immunity to dis-ease. Your *Wellness* develops as *you* develop a hardy personality with an optimistic, cheerful, friendly, and happy outlook on life. Sign the Wellness Contract.

Your illness begins in your mind. Strong and negative forces program and condition you to be ill. You have been conditioned and taught to think negatively, tolerate violence, eat unhealthily, accept air pollution, destruction of the forests, ruining of the sun's rays and acidificiation of the rain. You are programmed to accept the slaughter carried out by cigarette companies, alcohol manufacturers and the munitions industry. Thoughts are instilled in you that make you ill. 24% of the country's economy depends on it—12% makes you ill—12% repairs you when you are!

It is difficult to pay serious attention to these facts. You don't want to hear this because your *"Thinker"* rebels against it. For your life's sake, it is necessary to quiet your *"Thinker."* It is much more important for you to be happy than right. You *are* part of the most overweight, stressed out, gouty, hypertensive, arthritic, atherosclerotic, hemorrhoidal, ulcer ridden, cancer, coronary and stroke prone population in the world. *You are part of the most overmedicated, oversurgerized, overradiated population since the beginning of recorded history.*

The *way* out of the dis-ease maze you are in—
particularly if you are ill or if you are just *sick and
tired* of being sick and tired—the *way* to get from
"here to there" and to save a massive amount of
money too, is through the Prescription For Life.
It requires your personal responsibility, enhances
your self-value and generates reverence for life.
That's what health is all about.

Bibliography

Assagioli, R., *Psychosynthesis*, N.Y., Viking, 1965.

Benson, H., *The Relaxation Response*, N.Y., Morrow, 1975.

Bettelheim, B., *The Informed Heart*, N.Y., Free Prescot Glencoe, 1965.

Bloomfield, H. and Kory, R., Innerjoy, N.Y., Wyden, 1983.

Borysenko, J., *Minding The Body, Mending The Mind,* Reading, Addison Wesley, 1987

Bressler, D., and Trubo, R., *Free Yourself from Pain*, N.Y., Simon & Schuster, 1979.

Brown, B., *Supermind*, N.Y., Harpur, 1980.

Buber, M., *I and Thou*,N.Y., Charles Scribner's Sons, 1970.

Capra, F., *The Tao of Physics*, N.Y., Dell, 1977.

Carlson, R.J., *The End of Medicine*, N.Y., Wiley, 1975.

Cousins, N., *Anatomy of an Illness as Perceived by the Patient*, N.Y., Bantam, 1981.

Cousins, N., *The Healing Heart,* N.Y., Norton, 1983.

Diamond, H. & M., *Fit for Life*, N.Y., Warner Books, 1985, *Living Health*, N.Y., Warner Books, 1987.

Diamond, M., *A New Way of Eating*, N.Y.,Warner Books, 1987.

Dossey, L., *Beyond Illness*, Boulder, Shambala, 1984.

Dubos, R., *Mirage of Health*, N.Y., Harper & Row, 1971.

Dunbar, F., *Emotions and Bodily Changes*, N.Y., Columbia University Press, 1954.

Ferguson, M., *The Aquarian Conspiracy*, L.A., J. P. Tarcher, 1980.

Framingham Study, The, Washington, D.C., GPO section 101, 1968.

Frank, J.D., *The Faith that Heals*, The Johns Hopkins Medical Journal, 1975, 137, 127-131.

Frankl, V., *Man's Search for Meaning*, N.Y., Washington Square Press, 1985.

Fromm, E., *The Art of Loving*, N.Y., Harper, 1956.

Fuchs, V., *Who Shall Live?*, N.Y., Basic Books, 1975.

Gawain, S., *Creative Visualization*, Mill Valley, Whatever Publications, 1978.

Greben, S. *Loves Labour*, N.Y., Schocken Books, 1984.

Green, E., *Beyond Biofeedback*, N.Y., Delacorts, 1977.

Hesse, H., *Siddhartha*, N.Y., New Directions, 1957.

Hutschnecker, A., *The Will To Live*, N.Y., Crowell 1953; N.Y., Cornerstone Library, 1974.

Illich, I., *Medical Nemesis*, N.Y., Pantheon, 1976.

Inglefinger, F.J., *Health: A Matter of Statistics or Feeling*, New England Journal of Medicine, February 24, 1977, 448-449.

Jaffe, D.T., *Healing From Within*, N.Y., Bhataui, 1980.

James, W., *Psychology*, N.Y., World Publishing Company, 1948.

Jampolsky, G., *Love is Letting Go of Fear*, Berkeley, Celestial Arts, 1979.

Justice, B., *Who Gets Sick*, L.A., Tarcher, 1988.

Kapuchuk, T., Croucher, M., *The Healing Arts*, N.Y., Summit, 1987.

Krystal, P., *Cutting the Ties that Bind*, L.A., Aura Books, 1983.

Laing, R.D., *The Politics of Experience* N.Y., Ballantine Books, 1969.

Lappe, F., *Diet for a Small Planet*, N.Y., Ballantine, 1971.

La Laude, M., *A New Perspective on the Health of Canadians*, Ottawa, Canada, Minister of National Health and Welfare Information, 1975.

Le Boyer, F., *Birth Without Violence*, N.Y., Knopf, 1975.

LeShan, L., *How to Meditate*, N.Y., Bantam, 1974.

Levi, L., *Society Stress and Disease*, N.Y., Oxford University Press, 1971.

Locke, S., Colligan, D., *The Healer Within*, N.Y., Mentor, 1986.

Lowen, H., *The Language of the Body*, N.Y., Collier, 1971.

Maslow, A.H., *Toward A Psychology of Being*, N.Y., Nostrand, 1968.

Marti-Ilbanez, F., N.Y., Clarkson Potter, 1951.

Mason, V., *Practical Guide To Survival*, Orange, Mason/Slawson 1987.

Mendelsohn, R., *Male Practice,* Chicago, Contemporary Books, 1979.

Murphy, J., *The Power of the Subconscious Mind,* N.Y., Prentice Hall, 1963.

Nolen, W.H., *Surgeon Under the Knife,* N.Y., Dell, 1977.

O'Hara, V., *The Fitness Option,* La Jolla Stress Institute, 1988.

Osler, W., *Aequanimitas,* N.Y., McGraw-Hill 1906.

Owen, B., *Roger's Recovery from AIDs,* Malibu, Davar, 1987.

Oyle, I., *The Healing Mind,* N.Y., Pocket books, 1979.

Pion, R., *The Last Sex Manual,* N.Y., Wyden, 1977.

Peck, M.S., *The Road Less Travelled,* N.Y., Simon & Schuster, 1985.

Pellitier, K.R., *Mind as Healer, Mind as Slayer,* N.Y., Delacorte Press/Seymour Lawrence, 1977.

Penfield, W., *The Mystery of the Mind,* Princeton, N.J., Princeton University Press, 1975.

Salk, J., *Personal Communications.*

Sandweiss, S., *Spirit and Mind,* San Diego, Birthday Publishing, 1985.

Schweitzer, A., *Out of My Life and Thought,* An Autobiography, N.Y., 1949, Holt.

Selye, H., *Stress Without Distress,* N.Y., Dutton, 1974.

Siegel, B.S., *Love, Medicine & Miracles*, N.Y., Harper and Row, 1986.

Simonton, O.C., Matthews-Simonton, S. and Creighton, J., *Getting Well Again*, L.A., J.P. Tarcher, 1978.

Sontag, S., *Illness as Metaphor*, N.Y., Farrar, Straus & Giroux, 1978.

Szent-/Gyorgy, A., *Bioelectronics*, N.Y., Academic Press, 1968.

Taub, E. and A., *Health For Life*, Sausalito, American Wellness Association, 1989.

Thomas, L., *The Lives of a Cell*, N.Y., Bantam, 1975.

Tracy, L., *The Gradual Vegetarian*, N.Y., Dell, 1986.

Travis, J.W., *Wellness Workbook*, Mill Valley, Wellness Center, 1979.

Virchow, R., *Disease, Life, and Man*, Stanford, Stanford University Press, 1958.

Weed, L.L., *Medical Records, Medical Education, and Patient Care*, Chicago, Case Western Reserve University Press, 1970.

Wolf, F., *The Body Quantum*, N.Y., Macmillan, 1986.

Yogananda, P., *Autobiography of a Yogi*, L.A., Self Realization Fellowship, 1973.

Psychoneuroimmunology Bibliography

(Abstracted from a most comprehensive review of this topic by Kenneth R. Pellitier and Denise L. Herzing. In Volume 5, Number 1 of *Advances,* the Journal of the Institute for the Advancement of Health. The title of the paper is: Psychoneuroimmunology: Towards a mind body model.)

Ader R. *Psychoneuroimmunology.* New York: Academic Press, 1981.

Ader R. Development psychoneuroimmunology. *Dev Psychobiol* 1983; 16(4):251-67.

Ahlquist J. Hormonal influences on immunologic and related phenomena. In: Ader R. ed. *Psychoneuroimmunology.* New York: Academic Press, 1981, pp. 355-403.

Andrews G, Tennant C. Life event stress, social support, coping style and the risk of psychological impairment. *J. Nerv & Ment Dis* 1978;166(7): 605-12.

Bartrop RW, Lazarus L, Luckhurst E, Kiloh LG, Penny R. Depressed lymphocyte function after bereavement. *Lancet* 1977;1:834-6.

Besedovsky HO, del Rey AE, Sorkin E. What do the immune system and the brain know about each other? *Immunol Today* 1983;4(12):342-6.

Black S, Humphrey JH, Niven JS. Inhibition of mantoux reaction by direct suggestion under hypnosis. *Br Med J* 1963;6:1649-52.

Bloom B, Asher S, White S. Marital disruption as a stressor: A review and analysis. *Psychol Bull* 1978;85(6):867-94.

Borysenko M. Area review: Psychoneuroimmunology. *Ann Behav Med* 1987;9(2):3-10.

Boyce WT, Jensen EW, Cassel JC, Collier AM, Smith AH, Ramey CT. Influence of life events and family routines on childhood respiratory tract illness. *Pediatrics* 1977; 60:609-15.

Braun B. Psychophysiologic phenomena in multiple personality and hypnosis. *Am J Clin Hyp* 1983;26(2):124-37.

Chen E, Cobb S. Family structure in relation to health and disease. *J Chron Dis* 1960;12:544-67.

Cobb S, Kasl SV, French J, Norstebo G. The intrafamilial transmission of rheumatoid arthritis: Why do wives with rheumatoid arthritis have husbands with peptic ulcer? *J Chron Dis* 1969;22:279-93.

Cunningham A. Information and health in the many levels of man: Toward a more comprehensive theory of health and disease. *Advances* 1986;3(1):32-45.

Derogatis L, Abeloff M, Melisaratos N. Psycho-biological coping merchanisms and survival time in metastatic breast cancer. *JAMA* 1979;242:1504-8.

Dillon KM, Minchoff B, Baker KH. Positive emotional states and enhancement of the immune system. *Intl J Psychiat Med* 1985;-15:13-7.

Dossey L. Mind, medicine and the new physics: A time for re assessment. *Advances* 1988;5(1):- 57-69.

Earle JBB. Cerebral laterality and meditation: A review of the literature. *J Transpers Psychol* 1981;13(2):155-73.

Finke RA. Mental imagery and the visual system. *Scient Am* 1986;254(3):88-95.

Fox B. Psychosocial factors and the immune system in human cancer. In: Ader R., ed., *Psychoneuroimmunology.* New York: Academic Press, 1981, pp. 103-82.

Goodkin K, Antoni MH, Blaney PH. Stress and hopelessness in the promotion of cervical intraepithelial neoplasia to invasive squamous cell carcinoma of the cervix. *J Psychosom Res* 1986;30(1):67-76.

Jacobs MA, Spilken A, Norman M. Relationship of life change, maladaptive aggression, and upper respiratory infection in male college students. *Psychosom Med* 1969;31:31-44.

Kasl SV, Evans AS, Niederman JC. Psychosocial risk factors in the development of infectious mononucleosis. *Psychosom Med* 1979;41:445-66.

Keicolt-Glaser J, Garner W, Speicher C, Penn G, Holiday J, Glaser R. Psychosocial modifiers of immunocompetence in medical students. *Psychosom Med* 1984;46(1):7-14.

Keicolt-Glaser JK, Glaser R, Williger D, Stout JC, Tarr KL, Speicher CE. Psychosocial enhancement of immunocompetence in a geriatric population. *Health Psychol* 1985;4:25-41.

Kissen DM. Psychosocial factors, personality, and lung cancer in men aged 55-64. *Br J Med Psychol* 1967;40:29-43.

Kobasa SC. The hardy personality: Toward a social psychology of stress and health. In: Sanders GS, Suls J, eds., *Social psychology of health and illness.* Hillsdale, NJ: Lawrence Erlbaum, 1982.

Ley RG. Cerebral laterality and imagery. In: *Imagery: Current theory, research, and application.* New York: Wiley, 1983, pp. 69-86.

Libet B. Unconscious cerebral initiative and the role of conscious will in voluntary action. *Beh & Brain Sci* 1985;8:529-66.

Linn BS, Linn MW, Jensen J. Degree of depression and immune responsiveness. *Psychosom Med* 1982;44:128-9 (abstract).

Maslow A. Dynamics of personality organization. *Psychol Rev* 1943;50:514-58.

McClelland DC, Kirshnit C. The effect of motivational arousal through films on salivary immune function. Unpublished paper. Harvard University, 1984.

Ornstein R, Sobel D. The healing brain. *Psychol Today* March 1987;48-52.

Pelletier KR, Peper E. Alpha EEG feedback as a means for pain control. *J Clin & Exp Hyp* 1976;25(41):361-71.

Pert CB. The wisdom of the receptors: Neuropeptides, the emotions, and bodymind. *Advances* 1986;-3(3):8-16.

Pettingale KW, Morris T, Greer S. Mental attitudes to cancer: An additional prognostic factor. *Lancet* 1985;1:750.

Reite M, Harbeck R, Hoffman A. Altered cellular immune response following peer separation. *Life Sci* 1981;29:1133-6.

Schleifer S, Keller S, Cammerino M, Thornton J, Stein M. Suppression of lymphocyte stimulation following bereavement. *JAMA* 1983;250(3):374-7.

Seligman MEP. *Helplessness: On depression, development, and death.* San Francisco: Freeman, 1975.

Selye H. *The physiology and pathology of exposure to stress.* Montreal: Acta, 1975.

Silberman ED, Weingartner H. Hemispheric lateralization of functions related to emotion. *Brain & Cognition* 1986;5:322-53.

Smith GR, and McDaniel SM. Psychologicalty medicated effect on the delayed hypersensitivity reaction to tuberculin in humans. *Psychosomatic Medicine* 1983;45(1):65-70.

Solomon GF, Moos RH. Psychologic aspects of response to treatment in rheumatoid arthritis. *Gen Psychiat* 1965;114:113-9.

Solomon GF, Amkraut AA. Psychoneuroendocrinological effects of the immune response. *Annual Rev Microbiol* 1981;35:155-84.

Steiner H, Higgs CMB, Fritz GK, Laszlo G, Harvey JE. Defense style and the perception of asthma. *Psychosom Med* 1987;49(1):35-44.

Smith GR, McKenzie JM, Marmer DJ, Steele RW. Psychologic modulation of the human immune response to varicella zoster. *Arch Int Med.* 1985;145:2110-1.

Solomon GF. Emotional and personality factors in the onset and course of autoimmune disease, particularly rheumatoid arthritis. In: Ader R. Ed. *Psychoneuroimmunology.* New York: Academic Press, 1981.

Thomas CB, Drush A, Brown CH, Shaffer JW, Duszynski KR. Cancer in families of former medical students followed to mid-life-Prevalence in relatives of subjects with and without major cancer. *Johns Hopkins Med* 1982;151(5): 193-202.

Totman RG, Kiff J. Life stress and susceptibility to colds. In: Osborne D.J., Gruneberg M.M., Eiser JR. eds. *Research in psychology and medicine,* vol. 1. New York: Academic Press, 1979, p. 141-9.

About The Author

Edward A. Taub, M.D., has been engaged in the clinical practice of Medicine for twenty five years and is an Associate Clinical Professor at the University of California Medical School at Irvine. Dr. Taub wrote the historic foreword that introduced the book *"Fit for Life"* to over four million readers and is widely recognized for his pioneering work in the fields of patient self care and health care cost containment.

Dr. Taub conducts Voyage to Wellness seminars throughout the world on passenger ships including the Queen Elizabeth II, the Stardancer, the Vistafjord, the Sagafjord, and the Caribe. Prior to beginning his lecture series Dr. Taub worked with corporate and labor union leaders to develop and implement employee wellness programs designed to help reduce health care costs and absenteeism and promote efficiency on the job.

Dr. Taub is the Chairman of the American Wellness Association and the Founder of Integrative Medicine. As discussed in his book *"Prescription For Life,"* Integrative Medicine is a biosocial and psychospiritual approach to understanding health and dealing with disease based upon the concept that our health requires personal responsibility, self value, and reverence for life. Integrative Medicine advocates recognition of our own bodies natural abilities of self healing and involvement in our own health care as part of a physician-patient partnership.

Dr. Taub attended the Bronx H.S. of Science, Harpur College of the State University of New York. He received his medical degree from the Upstate Medical Center in Syracuse. Dr. Taub received training in psychiatry and medicine through the National Institutes of Health and completed his Pediatric Residency at the Los Angeles General Hospital Medical Center of the University of Southern California.

Dr. Taub served as a Lieutenant Commander in the United States Public Health Service, and was the first Wellness Director for the Organized Labor (AFL-CIO/Teamsters) Movement. He is a frequent guest lecturer at Universities, Institutes and Medical Meetings and founded the Tustin-Irvine Pediatric Medical Group, the Alta Institute of Integrative Medicine and the Foundation for Health Awareness.

Dr. Taub is a member of the American Medical Association, a Diplomate of the National Board of Medical Examiners, a Fellow of the American Academy of Pediatrics, a New York Regents Scholar, a Clark Foundation Scholar and a Wyeth Fellow. He is the President of the Integrative Medicine Institute.